M000189932

C. DIFF

CLOSTRIDIUM DIFFICILE
AND COLITIS

oils for circulation

Ginger, Cypress
* Eucalyptus dialtor
Coriander topically

a) Wintergreen thin blood?
Juniper removes uric
Blk pepper Acid Crystals
Disp) Dissolve cholesterol
Lavender
relieve anxiety
Cumin pain

More books by Ellen Pendleton:

Read & Run
Take A Hike
Write On!

The Grandma Camping books:
Little Tree
Grace, Gophers, & Garlic
Arbolito / Little Tree
My First Camping Trip

C. DIFF

CLOSTRIDIUM DIFFICILE AND COLITIS

by

ELLEN PENDLETON

espbooks

espbooks.net
CARMEL CALIFORNIA USA

C. DIFF

CLOSTRIDIUM DIFFICILE
AND COLITIS

by ELLEN PENDLETON

International Standard Book Number 978-0-9815428-2-9
International Standard Book Number 0-9815428-2-4

Previously published as *Clostridium difficile and Colitis: A Personal Journey*

http://www.CDIFFbook.com

First Edition
Published by *espbooks.net*
P.O. Box 221238
Carmel CA 93922 USA
espbooks@gmail.com

Printed in USA by CreateSpace.com

~ Dedicated to you ~

Be well

and

Trust your Gut!

DISCLAIMER

I am not a medical expert or doctor, nor do I have medical education. I am not an investigative journalist. This is not a self-help book, how-to book, or instructions. I am not writing this to chastise or take revenge on the periodontist that did the work or Western Medicine as an entity. This book is not advice.

ENTER AT YOUR OWN RISK

This book is autobiographical, my personal journey, a journal of the resources that I found along the way, most of them from the Internet. I am a writer who would rather be backpacking, traveling, camping or writing about backpacking and travel adventures, than dealing with health issues.

I followed my intuition, my inner guru, to recover my well-being. If you have been diagnosed with Toxigenic *C. difficile* and colitis may this book help to expedite your recovery by providing Internet links of information, experience and hope.

I write this book with the dream that what happened to me will never happen to another Spirit Being Human here on Planet Earth.

I never know what I think about something until I read what I've written on it.
— William Faulkner

Contents

~ BEING WELL ~

procrastinate, *v.i.;* procrastinated, *pl., pp.;* procrastinating, *ppr.* [from L. *procrastinatus,* pp. of *procrastinare; pro,* for, forward, and *crastinus,* belonging to the morrow, from *cras,* tomorrow.] to put off doing something until a future time; to postpone or defer taking action.

Life is good. I took an early social security retirement last year so I could have time to travel, write and go backpacking in the Sierra, my passions. I am mother of three grown children and have three beautiful grandchildren who are growing up way too quickly.

I am an amateur athlete and a retired hiking guide. My education and work was in electronics. I also worked as an associate editor and a dessert chef.

At age 43, I began backpacking in the Sierra Nevada Range of Light in California and absolutely fell in love with it. At age 45 I began backpacking solo in the Sierra and writing books about it. At age 49, I trained and ran the Big Sur International Marathon as a result of a deal with my boss. Having never been a runner I took training seriously and did well, 4:11. At 50 I ran across

1

the Grand Canyon rim-to-rim on a last minute whim. At age 51 I ran around the island of Rarotonga in the Cook Islands, just for fun. My children call hiking with me *Ellen's Death March*. My little ones call me *Grandma Camping*.

This last August, age 62, and this is where *procrastination* comes in, I took a month-long solo backpacking trek from southern Sequoia National Park, California, north to Red's Meadow near Mammoth, visiting the three primitive hot springs (that I know) along the way. I have yet to finish writing that book. It will come. The trip was awesome, all was well, fit as a fiddle, blah, blah, blah. But I have a tooth that needs attention and I put it off until after the trip.

To make a short story long I waited too long and now it is not to be saved. Okay, I don't mind rattlesnakes and bears but I really don't like going to the dentist. My bad. It hurts. I make an appointment with a local periodontist who specializes in implants.

1 December, Monday
Pre-Appointment Paperwork

Whenever you find yourself on the side of the majority, it is time to pause and reflect.
— Mark Twain

I go to the dentist office to fill out the paperwork and get ready for tomorrow's appointment. I sit with an office person who gives me the options and the corresponding fees. She also gives the pre-appointment instructions and a prescription.

"What is this?" I ask.

"This is a prescription for an antibiotic to take as a preventative," she returns.

I wrinkle my face and look her in the eyes.

"It is *standard protocol*," she defends.

"I'm allergic to penicillin."

"We see that on your paperwork and this one is okay for penicillin allergies."

Okay, whatever. I just want this tooth out the easiest way possible. I go to Pharmaca and get the prescription filled, then next door to Trader Joe's for post-procedure soft foods.

2 DECEMBER, TUESDAY
TOOTH EXTRACTION

When everyone is thinking the same, no one is thinking.
— John Wooden, UCLA basketball coach

I go to my dentist appointment eager to have this tooth gone. He tries his best to talk me out of extraction, wanting to save the tooth. I settle on letting him put ground up bone in the tooth hole to hopefully grow with my jaw bone. Then later, he can put in an implant having something to work with. Whatever, just take this tooth out. I want it gone. I expect this to be an easy fix. I want this tooth out. I want to be rid of it. This is all I can think of.

The procedure takes longer than I want, I get cold and start shaking. I am afraid. Childhood memories of our sadistic family dentist come up. I remember sitting in the chair, mouth open, unable to talk, scream, move, fight or resist and he'd drill away with an evil grin on his face. My mom didn't believe me or didn't care. Nightmare.

Finally, the tooth is out and they pack it with someone else's ground up bone that makes me feel creepy. Enough therapy. I give them my credit card and they ring up $1622.00. I take my pretty blue party bag full of gauze, mouthwash, Vicodin, Ibuprofen, Post Treatment Instructions, precautions and make the drive home. My cupboard is full of applesauce, boxed soups, juices, non-dairy milks, protein powder, electrolytes and hope.

The after-surgery pain continues as expected when the novocaine wears off and I start in on the Vicodin 5/325, taking only half every 4-6 hours. Doc also packaged up Ibuprofen 400 mg #20 with instructions to TAKE ONE TABLET EVERY 4-6 HOURS UNTIL GONE. I am little. I weigh about 110 pounds. I am fit, in shape, on no medications, no health issues, very active, hiking routinely but had a bad tooth.

Two-and-a-half years ago I changed to a whole

food, plant-based diet from reading Dr. John McDougall's book, *The Starch Solution* and watching the film, *Forks Over Knives*. With those two resources I immediately changed my diet and have not turned back. Then I read *The China Study* by T. Colin Campbell. It was an easy transition. The whole food, plant-based diet cookbooks available now are amazing and full of exciting, incredible recipes and ideas. I'd been a vegan before but this time was different because the cookbooks, websites and support made all of the difference. Before it was, *can't eat this, can't eat that.* But now it is really an adventure to try new cooking techniques and recipes. The diet does not include any oil: olive oil, coconut oil, canola oil, no oil. I sauté with water. Standard American Diet, SAD, has ruled our tastebuds and it is a change to leave animal flesh, butter, olive oil, sugar, milk, cheese and eggs behind. But the trade-off is well worth it.

So I am ready to weather the storm, heal my mouth and be on with it.

5 December, Friday

Just listen to your body, eat in silence and see what feels good and you will spontaneously choose the foods that are beneficial to you.
— Deepak Chopra

My inner guru says, "Stop taking this," referring to the antibiotic that I've been taking, sensing it is not in my body's best interest. I have taken 12 of the 21 pills. I listen to my inner guidance and stop.

~ THEN LIFE CHANGED ~

16 DECEMBER, TUESDAY

The dentist removes the sutures.

19 DECEMBER, FRIDAY

I don't feel well but force myself to go out to a holiday art gathering. I eat dinner before going out because I am so picky about my diet and I'm still on kind of a soft diet. Usually these gatherings have a lot of cheese, crackers, chips and chocolate, the four Cs. My gut feels a bit weird but I go.

I eat three small pieces of celery at the party, (another "C" food).

When we get home, my gut is upset but why? Dinner was fine but the celery isn't settling well. How could that be?

I have a couple of girlfriends who are like, healing. We take care of each other. They know when I need to be taken care of.
— Maggie Gyllenhaal

What? Diarrhea all day. About ten stools. I spend the day in the bathroom. I don't want to take anything for it but just let it run its course. I drink some rice milk and lots of water. We plan to go to a party tonight but I really don't feel like going.

EMAIL
LEENDA

I am having intestinal issues and have spent most of the day in the potty room. Just thought you wanted this information. Humph.

No clue why.

ellen
END EMAIL

I am spent. If I go to the party tonight I worry that I'll spend most of my time in the bathroom. I feel crappy (excuse the pun) but rally up to go. It's a friend's annual pot luck Christmas party and the usual suspects will be there; people we sometimes see only once a year at this party. It's a tribal event.

Again, I eat before we go knowing how picky I am about food. My other whole, Claudio, knows what a day I had, so I make a plan: "I might need to bow out, go to the car and I might not be able to tell you first. I'll take the spare car key. If I leave the party I will go to the car. Don't worry about me just party on. I'll have my cell phone. If you can't find me, call." Claudio suggests some PeptoBismo but I decline.

Sure enough the table is full of cheese, salmon, sugar, oily salads and lamb. I bring freshly cut pineapple, eat some and a bit of cantaloup. My gut feels crampy and I don't have any energy to stand and talk so I sit near the piano and listen to the music all night. People come by, sit and visit. I make it through the party without incident.

When we get home, the diarrhea begins again.

EMAIL
Ln
Oh no! Are you picking up stuff being the empath that you are? Do you want me to bring you charcoal?

Linda
END EMAIL

EMAIL TO LEENDA
I forgot about charcoal. Thanks for the reminder. I have some. Good idea. I felt funny emailing you regarding this but you pulled through with a GREAT recommendation. BRAVO, Goddess of Intuition.

ellen
END EMAIL

I take some charcoal, wait an hour and take some grapefruit seed extract.

>> On Dec 20, 2014, at 21:01, Linda wrote:

>> Ln

>> How are you feeling?

>> Did you go out to the

>> Party?

>> I wandered around after the family dinner! I like to walk the streets around here.

>> There is a kind of clay that

>> works to help bind poop if you are still having issues.

END EMAIL

EMAIL

> On Dec 21, 2014, at 12:31 AM, espbooks@gmail.com wrote:

> LEENDA

> Just got home from the party. Didn't have any messy mishaps. Whew! I am good. Thanks.

>

> Bedtime

> ellen

END EMAIL

21 DECEMBER, SUNDAY

EMAIL

On Dec 21, 2014 at 11:21 AM, Linda wrote:

Glad no more messy mishaps.

LEENDA

END EMAIL

The abdominal cramps intensify and really hurt. The diarrhea continues every hour or so through the night.

22 December, Monday

I don't have time for this. Christmas is coming and I will be cooking dinner for the family and taking it to my daughter's house for the celebration. I have shopping to do and presents to wrap. I cannot leave the house. The diarrhea continues every hour or so all day and through the night with abdominal cramps.

23 December, Tuesday

More of the same. Claudio takes me grocery shopping. I know where the restrooms are in all of the grocery stores.

I'm glad to be home again. I work and poo!

Again the diarrhea continues about every hour and through the night. I am exhausted.

24 December, Wednesday

The abdominal cramps really hurt. The diarrhea runs its course but now whenever I go to the toilet, mucous balls come out. I am all out of poo. I have no appetite, have lost weight and I'm very tired.

I run my course too, cooking dinner for all. It is my JOY and pleasure to cook and be with my BELOVED for Christmas Eve and we all have a grand time. My grandbabies are growing up. The youngest is ten. So big but not too big for Santa.

Claudio goes to his ex's house to have Christmas dinner with his grown children and invites me to join him. I am having gut cramps and just want to go home. He leaves.

Fortunately, the mucous balls wait until I leave the party to begin again. I mess my panties on the way home. Disgusting.

I am up and down all night, leaving the bathroom light on since I am in there so often. I went potty at least twenty times today. I do not sleep.

~ KEYWORDS ~

25 DECEMBER, THURSDAY

You shall know the truth and the truth shall make you mad.
— Aldous Huxley

Christmas morning. I weigh in at 104.2 pounds, a little light for me. I like 110 pounds. Last night I went to the potty almost every hour, so I didn't sleep well. I feel awful. Maybe some rice milk will slow down the mucous balls; no poo left. I remember a product I used to have, a powder made from brown rice, that worked well to stop diarrhea.

11

DIARR–EASE, or something like that. I drink some rice milk. I don't have an appetite. I feel weak and stay in bed except for potty breaks.

I get on the laptop and KEYWORD in the symptoms: **DIARRHEA, MUCOUS STOOLS, WEIGHT LOSS, FATIGUE.** Much to my surprise, IRRITABLE BOWEL SYNDROME (IBS) comes up. I remember Mickel Therapy: *What was going on in your life when you first started noticing symptoms?* is the question. Yes, I had some stressful family issues at the time I noticed symptoms but I really don't feel that my symptoms stem from emotional stress. Not this time. This is not a software problem. This is a hardware issue. The tooth extraction was stressful. My thoughts travel. Does the Post Treatment Instruction handout mention diarrhea? Antibiotic. What antibiotic did I take? I get out of bed to find the container.

Clindamycin HCl 300 mg Cap Ranb. ONE CAPSULE BY MOUTH THREE TIMES A DAY WITH FOOD UNTIL GONE.

Okay, but my sense was to stop taking it, so I did. I go to the Internet to look up the adverse side effects of clindamycin.

****

Clindamycin HCl Side Effects
http://www.ehow.com/about_4745364_clindamycin-hcl-side-effects.html **By Shelley Moore, eHow Contributor**
****

Colitis can be a side effect? What is colitis?
****

Causes of Colitis

- Colitis can result from antibiotic treatment because these agents kill friendly bacteria as well, permitting overgrowth of the drug-resistant *clostridia*, which produces a toxin that causes colitis. The severe type of colitis seen with clindamycin HCl treatment, called pseudomembranous colitis, can almost always be eliminated with other antibiotics. However, in rare cases, the condition requires removal of the colon, or may even be fatal.

Warning

- Clindamycin HCl can cause a severe type of colitis, an intestinal disease resulting from a form of resistant bacteria. The disease may even occur months after treatment has ended. Patients should contact their doctor immediately if they begin suffering from abdominal cramps, continued diarrhea, or bloody stools. They should not use anti-diarrhea or narcotic pain medicine, because these actually can make the symptoms worse.

****

WTF????!!!!! Excuse me? An adverse side effect could be removal of my colon or death???

I ask my computer, What is pseudomembranous colitis? The search offers many choices and I go with Wikipedia. The pseudomembranous colitis redirects to:

****

http://en.wikipedia.org/wiki/Clostridium_difficile_colitis

****

OMG ~ It's not the diarrhea, the colectomy surgery or the dying that bothers me; this is what hits me the hardest: It causes an **infectious** diarrhea. Overgrowth of Clostridium difficile (a bacteria) can cause this diarrhea.

13

INFECTIOUS!!!!!!! I cooked Christmas dinner for my beautiful children and my beautiful grandbabies. OMG!!! If I have been infectious and if I have given them this horrible thing, ... This would kill me. I have been cooking dinner at home for me, Claudio and sometimes my brother Tom, when he visits. I read on.

****

Okay, I have these symptoms: *Significant diarrhea ("new onset of more than three partially formed or watery stools per 24-hour period"), recent antibiotic exposure, abdominal pain, ...*

I have been going poo twenty times in 24 hours! That is more that three. I have been living on the toilet. Lemme dig out the dentist's instructions and cautions. Periodontal Therapy Post Treatment Instructions. Number 4 . . . *In case you should develop a skin rash, diarrhea or nausea, stop taking the antibiotic and call our office.*

I have diarrhea. I should call the doctor.

It is 10 a.m. Christmas morning and he has two Little Ones, twin boys. The Post Treatment Instructions say: *For the convenience of our patients the Doctor or a live member of the team is on call even after hours for any urgent needs you may have post surgery, by calling PHONE # . . . .*

****

I read more about antibiotic-induced colitis and C.

difficile and there it is: Clindamycin.

Probiotics. I should have been taking probiotics. I rarely take antibiotics and I forgot about backing it up with probiotics. Too bad the doc didn't recommend probiotics. I have some old probiotics in the refrigerator and I take a couple.

****

http://en.wikipedia.org/wiki/Clostridium_difficile_colitis

Drugs used to slow or stop diarrhea such as loperamide may worsen *C.difficile* disease, so are not recommended.[49] Cholestyramine, an ion exchange resin, is effective in binding both toxin A and B, slowing bowel motility, and helping prevent dehydration.[50]

http://en.wikipedia.org/wiki/Loperamide = Imodium
http://en.wikipedia.org/wiki/Clostridium_difficile_colitis
NOTE: See online for research footnote list.
This link has a twelve-page research footnote section and reading all of these links may take a while. Hours of entertainment.

****

I am concerned. This is infectious and I am the cook here.

Writing helps me clarify the chaos. I intend to beat this, recover my well-being and journal through the entire process. I trust that I will feel well enough to go backpacking this season and walk the *Camino de Santiago* in France and Spain next year. I have things to do and places to go.

As Spirits Being Human here on Planet Earth, the first step in getting well is being at peace with Body,

Mind and Spirit, trusting the inner guidance, *inner guru* or *guru within.* TRUST is huge. I LOVE life and I am not finished adventuring and exploring this gorgeous Planet Earth.

~ THE DANGEROUS PHONE CONVERSATION ~

I call the doc, make it through the automated answering system and, much to my surprise, the doctor answers. "Hello?"

"Hello DDS - This is Ellen Pendleton. I apologize for calling you Christmas morning but I am having a post-treatment issue of great concern."

"Okay, what is going on?"

"Well, I had a tooth extracted December 2 and took the antibiotic, clindamycin. I quit taking it after four days. On December 16th you took the sutures out and soon after I started getting gut issues that turned into diarrhea. I was having about twenty stools a day. Now I am just passing mucous balls. My fear is that I might have antibiotic-induced pseudomembranous colitis and *Clostridium difficile* bacteria."

"*CDIFF* is very rare. I doubt that you have it. Do

you have a family doctor?"

"No, I don't. I usually don't need one. I am healthy."

"Do you have a fever?" he asks.

"I don't know."

"Do you still have diarrhea?"

"Yes."

"Now, . . . it's a home remedy but black tea could stop the diarrhea. And you could take some Imodium. Do you have any Imodium?"

I pause, wrinkle my face and say, "But what if I have *Clostridium difficile* bacteria? I read that one should not take any anti-diarrhea medications, especially Imodium, because with *Clostridium difficile* it could make things worse."

"*C. difficile* is very rare. I doubt that you have it. Take your temperature and call me back, . . . not right away, . . . in a couple of hours, and let me know if you have a fever. Okay?"

"Okay."

Black tea stops diarrhea? I have never heard of this.

I get out of bed to find the thermometer. I look and look but cannot find it. I call the closest store to see if they are open. It's Christmas Day. Yes. Claudio goes to buy a thermometer. I fix a cup of tea.

17

Soon after Claudio leaves I find the thermometer and take my temperature: 95.2 degrees. No fever. That's a bit lower than normal, however. What is that all about?

I wait awhile to call back the doctor, letting him have his time with his Little Ones and hoping the black tea will work.

I go back into the world wide web to learn more:
****
From the National Institute of Health
http://www.nlm.nih.gov/medlineplus/druginfo/meds/a682399.html
Clindamycin
pronounced as (klin" da mye' sin)
IMPORTANT WARNING:
Many antibiotics, including clindamycin, may cause overgrowth of dangerous bacteria in the large intestine. This may cause mild diarrhea or may cause a life-threatening condition called colitis (inflammation of the large intestine). Clindamycin is more likely to cause this type of infection than many other antibiotics, so **it should only be used to treat serious infections that cannot be treated by other antibiotics.** Tell your doctor if you have or have ever had colitis or other conditions that affect your stomach or intestines.

You may develop these problems during your treatment or up to several months after your treatment has ended. Call your doctor if you experience any of the following symptoms during your treatment with clindamycin or during the first several months after your treatment has finished: watery or bloody stools, diarrhea, stomach cramps, or fever.
Talk to your doctor about the risks of taking clindamycin.
****

Oh great! Why didn't I question this earlier? Why did I just believe the "Standard Protocol" and trust the doc? If

I would have read the adverse side effects of clindamycin before I took it, I might not have taken it. And I did not have an infection. I was very healthy! It was a preventative.

****

Imodium: http://www.rxlist.com/imodium-drug/overdosage-contraindications.htm ~ **CONTRAINDICATIONS** ~ in patients with pseudomembranous colitis associated with the use of broad- spectrum antibiotics.

http://www.rxlist.com/script/main/art.asp?articlekey=5099
Pseudomembranous colitis: Severe inflammation of the inner lining of the colon. Pseudomembranous colitis is characterized by pus and blood in the stool and often caused by antibiotics.

****

1:30 p.m. I call the doctor back. He's glad to hear that I don't have a fever and the diarrhea has seemed to slow.

"Okay. I recommend that since you don't have a doctor, go to an Urgent Care type facility as soon as you can for lab tests. I am glad to hear that the black tea might be working. Please call back and update me. Okay?"

"Can you request lab tests?"

"No. That's out of my practice. I can't write this up. You'll have to go to another doctor."

"Okay."

I go online. I prefer the Urgent Care near Fisherman's Wharf but since my insurance was cancelled four months before ObamaCare took over, I had to change my insurance and Urgent Care doesn't take it. I find a

Doctors on Duty in New Monterey near Cannery Row. They are closed today. I drink more tea, sit in bed doing more Internet searching and get out my natural healing books.

Yesterday I had never heard the words *colitis*, *Clostridium difficile*, and *clindamycin*. Today I am in another world. Oh my.

~ LAB TESTING ~

I look up the three antibiotics recommended to treat *C. difficile*: Metronidazole (Flagyl), vancomycin, Fidaxomicin.

****

Metronidazole~(Flagyl)
http://en.wikipedia.org/wiki/Metronidazole ~ *Due to its potential carcinogenic properties, metronidazole is banned in the European Union and the USA for veterinary use in the feed of animals and is banned for use in any food animals in the USA.[22][23]*

****

That's enough for me.

****

Vancomycin
http://en.wikipedia.org/wiki/Vancomycin
Common adverse drug reactions (≥1% of patients) associated

with IV vancomycin include: local pain, which may be severe, and thrombophlebitis.

Rare adverse effects (<0.1% of patients) include: anaphylaxis, toxic epidermal necrolysis, erythema multiforme, red man syndrome, superinfection, thrombocytopenia, neutropenia, leukopenia, tinnitus, and dizziness and/or ototoxicity.[6]

Vancomycin can induce platelet-reactive antibodies in the patient, leading to severe thrombocytopenia and bleeding with florid petechial hemorrhages, ecchymoses, and wet purpura.[13]

****

My odds are not so good these days.

****

Fidaxomicin
http://www.dificid.com
Adverse side effects:
http://www.dificid.com/downloads/Dificid_PI.pdf

****

Fidaxomicin looks about even with vancomycin as far as side effects but the recurrence/relapse percentage is lower with the Fidaxomicin.

****

My need to go to the toilet has lessened. Good tea, eh? Trader Joe's Spicy Chai with a monkey on the box. I sweeten it with powdered stevia and some almond milk. I make myself eat something: Mashed potatoes, Spicy Black Bean soup in a box, carrot juice with chia seeds.

I try to get some sleep.

26 DECEMBER, FRIDAY
URGENT CARE

Good food is wise medicine.
— Alison Levitt M.D.

Slept better last night not getting up every hour to go to the toilet. What to eat for breakfast? Who would have thunk that black tea would stop diarrhea? No mucous balls either. I eat more probiotics and some Spicy Black Bean soup. I shower and get ready to go to Doctors on Duty in Monterey.

Claudio drives.

At Doctors on Duty I am given a clipboard, pen and a stack of forms to fill out. The waiting room is full. I hear some hacking/coughing and look for a seat far away from the sound. It'll be about a two-and-a-half hour wait. I check in and do the paperwork, etc. and Claudio leaves to go anywhere else but here. When paperwork check-in is done, I take a walk. Two blocks away is a CVS drug store. Probiotics. I feel like I need some probiotics. It feels like it takes me forever to get two blocks. I am weak. I find some CVS brand probiotic pearls, 30 pearls, 15 billion whatever units probiotics come in, for under eleven dollars. I'm in. I also find an unsweetened ice tea. Tannin. Is it the tannin that stops the diarrhea? I take one of the probiotics and down it with the tea. Slowly I walk back to the urgent care facility to sit and wait.

This is surreal.

My turn arrives. The young assistant takes all of my vitals but I forget to note my blood pressure and weight. The doctor appreciates that I've been doing my homework. I tell him the whole story about the clindamycin, the diarrhea, the mucous balls and the suspected *Clostridium difficile*. He examines me, pokes my abdomen and writes up the lab test request. I am not sure what it all means but these are checked off on the lab test request:

ORGAN/DISEASE PANELS — Comp metabolic panel w/eGFR;
HEMOTOLOGY — CBC w/DIFF;
OTHER TESTS — C-Reactive protein;
STOOL PATHOGENS — Culture, stool, O & P w/permanent stain.

Hand-written in at the bottom is "**37212** *C. Dificile* **Toxin A & B TF**", circled, with *difficile* misspelled and a capital "D".

The doc recommends the BRAT diet: Bananas, Rice, Applesauce, and Tea. Okay, I can do that.

I gather my things and return to the front desk. They ask me to sign-off on the paperwork and give me more forms to fill out regarding who to contact in case I am disabled or dead. This is encouraging. I don't fill these out and choose to take them home and *maybe* bring back. They made a few mistakes on my medical history and we unsuccessfully try to correct it. I am tired and out of energy without any patience or fight left in me. I give it a "whatever."

Claudio and I drive to the lab. No other patients are waiting so I go right in. Blood tests and three little plastic take-home containers for stool samples. Whoopee.

Then comes the grocery stop at Trader Joe's. We buy a gallon of aloe juice, bananas, applesauce, green juice, potatoes and sweet potatoes. The mashed potatoes tasted really good yesterday. I LOVE to steam the organic Gold Yukon potatoes then dip into tahini. Next door at Pharmaca I buy six bottles of Kevita®, a sparkling probiotic drink sweetened with stevia. This feels good. I drink one and eat a banana. I am spent, eager to get home and in bed.

I have Christmas dinner leftovers in the fridge, (vegan Chile Rellenos and Cornbread Stuffing that are not on my BRAT diet) and have no appetite.

Home. I warm up the mashed potatoes and sprinkle with garlic powder, which is an antibacterial, I believe. I'll look it up. I set my iPod timer for one hour to let the mashed potatoes digest before I put anything else into my poor little gut. Next comes carrot juice with chia seeds, letting them soak about 15 minutes to soften. Again, I set the timer to let it digest before putting anything else down there. Mono eating, I shall call it. More Spicy Chai black tea. Take a break.

Food becomes the goal for the day. I need fuel and strength. Food for the rest of the day includes a banana, aloe, TJs Lemon Honey Echinacea juice with drops of cayenne tincture, brown rice w/cinnamon and some applesauce. No diarrhea. No bowel movements at all. Am I *empty? Eat and sleep. That's the best that I can do today.*

Ln
Are you feeling better?
Do you need me to bring you supplies?
Linda

hola

I spent the afternoon at Docs on Duty.
Dec 1 took clindamycin HCL as a preventative for some dental work. Had the dental work Dec 2. Stopped taking clindamycin after four days (my body didn't like it). Dec 16 Dr. took sutures out. Dec 19 diarrhea began and then the mucous joined in. I made it through Christmas, abdominal cramps and all. Yesterday i was down, down. Finally did some Internet research and figured out the connection with the dentist and the clindamycin HCl.

Christmas morning (yesterday) i called the periodontist. He offered two suggestions to stop the diarrhea: Black tea and Imodium. Fortunately I'd read that if the intestinal bacteria *Clostridium difficile* is present in the gut flora, then the Imodium would most likely make the colitis worse, lead to surgical intervention and possibly death. I told him this and he said that "*C. diff* is very rare and you probably don't have it."

I sent Claudio to the store for a thermometer and made a cup of tea, . . . and another.

So to make a short story long the diarrhea has stopped after drinking the black tea. Of course, I did not take the Imodium. It's a good thing I'd done some homework and didn't trust him.

Got some aloe, bananas, electrolytes, miso, applesauce, Latin Black Bean soup in a box, carrot juice and chia seeds.

whew

That's the deal.

Thank you for your concern and info
ellen
END EMAIL

EMAIL
Ln
I am glad the poop stopped. Anti-biotic's
responsible for mucous too?Crazy!

spinach good in miso soup
Linda
END EMAIL

EMAIL
LEENDA
Yes. Colitis. Inflammation of the colon. Gut on FIRE!! The
clindamycin HCl is a broad-spectrum antibiotic and may have killed
my delicate intestinal flora. The stool testing will tell if the *C.difficile*
bacteria has moved in, which is listed on the clindamycin side
effects insert. It's a gut gang war.

Now that the flood has stopped flowing i have to wait for a sample.
Wish me luck.

I am glad the gut wrench part has minimized.
Whew, what a day.

Too much info, eh?
Any advice or recommendations?

ellen
END EMAIL

27 DECEMBER, SATURDAY

*We need to give each other the space to grow, to be ourselves, to
exercise our diversity. We need to give each other space so that we may*

both give and receive such beautiful things as ideas, openness, dignity, joy, healing, and inclusion.
— Max de Pree

My bowels cooperate and the lab is open until 1 pm. Weird looking poo, mucous covered. Yuck. I hope I never have to do this again. I don't have any issues digging a hole and going poo out in the wilderness when I am backpacking, but putting them into little plastic containers and a paper bag is gross. Claudio drives us over to the lab in Monterey for the drop off. Done.

Home and back to bed. No energy. Today's food is much the same eating mono: Probiotics, aloe w/lime juice, applesauce, Spicy Chai black tea with freeze-dried calcium magnesium (ABCalm®), banana, Kevita, mashed potatoes, green juice. I spend all day in bed, reading and sleeping.

~ How Shall I Heal? ~

28 December, Sunday
Heal

Although the world is full of suffering, it is also full of the overcoming of it. — Helen Keller

I remember a VHS video series by Dr. Richard Schulze about *incurable* diseases and conditions of human health that provide important clues for recovery. We still have the series. I find it and it is called, *The Sam Biser Save Your Life Herbal Video Collection*, produced by The University of Natural Healing, Inc., a collection of rare videos on advanced natural healing techniques for supposedly incurable health conditions.

We have volumes five through twelve. I pop one into the VCR, get about 10 seconds of video and it stops, stuck in the VHS/DVD player. I fish it out and wind it up. I do it again and the same thing happens. I pick a different tape. One more time. Repeat. Damn.

I go online to see if the series is available on DVD and fail to find it. On Dr. Schulze's website https://www.herbdoc.com a free book is offered: *The Incurables*, and I call to order it.

EMAIL
Good morning LEENDA

5 plant-based probiotics:
http://www.onegreenplanet.org/vegan-health/5-plant-based-foods-packed-with-probiotics/
Sauerkraut, miso, coconut water kefir, kimchi, kombucha.
here's a vegan mango lassi made with coconut milk kefir:
http://www.onegreenplanet.org/vegan-food/recipe-mango-lassi/

have you ever made sauerkraut???

ellen

****

http://www.onegreenplanet.org/vegan-food/all-you-need-to-know-about-kombucha-learn-how-to-make-it
How to make Kombucha
****

http://www.onegreenplanet.org/author/Annie_Oliverio
Another, same website:
http://www.onegreenplanet.org/vegan-food/how-to-make-kombucha/
How to Make Kombucha by Annie Oliverio
****

Good article on vegan protein:
http://www.onegreenplanet.org/vegan-health/10-vegan-foods-packed-with-protein/

http://jac.oxfordjournals.org/content/51/6/1339.full.pdf
Antibiotics and hospital-acquired *Clostridium difficile*-associated diarrhoea: a systematic view

http://emedicine.medscape.com/article/186458-treatment
Faten N Aberra, MD, MSCE Assistant Professor Of Medicine, Division of Gastroenterology, Hospital of the University of Pennsylvania, University of Pennsylvania School of Medicine

Approach Considerations

The decision to treat *C. difficile* infection (CDI) and the type of therapy administered depend on the severity of infection, as well as the local epidemiology and type of *C. difficile* strains present. Except for perioperative prophylaxis, it is recommended that use of cephalosporin and clindamycin be restricted for infection prevention.
****

Definition of *perioperative prophylaxis* ~
http://en.wikipedia.org/wiki/Antibiotic_prophylaxis

Antibiotic prophylaxis refers to the prevention of <u>infection complications</u> using <u>antimicrobial therapy</u> (most commonly antibiotics).

An estimated 5 to 10 percent of hospitalized patients undergoing <u>otolaryngology</u> ("head and neck") surgery acquire a <u>nosocomial</u> ("hospital") infection, which adds a substantial cost and an average of 4 extra days to the hospital stay.[*citation needed*]

<u>http://medical-dictionary.thefreedictionary.com/perioperative</u>
Perioperative ~ The perioperative period, less commonly spelled the peroperative period, is the time period describing the duration of a patient's surgical procedure; this commonly includes ward admission, anesthesia, surgery, and recovery. Perioperative generally refers to the three phases of surgery: preoperative, intraoperative, and postoperative. The goal of perioperative care is to provide better conditions for patients before operation, during operation, and after operation.[1]

<u>http://medical-dictionary.thefreedictionary.com/Prophylaxis</u>
Prophylaxis ~ Prevention of or protective treatment for disease.
****
Back to:
<u>http://emedicine.medscape.com/article/186458-treatment</u>
No treatment is necessary for asymptomatic carriers.

In patients with severe or complicated CDI, oral vancomycin is recommended as first-line therapy due to faster symptom resolution and fewer treatment failures than when metronidazole is used.

Surgical intervention
Patients with fulminant colitis and toxic megacolon may require operative intervention, such as colectomy with preservation of the rectum. These patients' serum lactate levels and peripheral leukocyte counts may aid in the decision to operate; there is a

significant risk for perioperative mortality with elevated serum lactate levels (5 mmol/L) and leukocytosis (50,000 cells/μL). For more information, see the Medscape Reference articles Toxic Megacolon and Pseudomembranous Colitis Surgery.
****

Toxic Megacolon ~ What is this???

****

http://www.ncbi.nlm.nih.gov/pmc/articles/PMC2999149/

Toxic megacolon associated *Clostridium difficile* colitis.

Sayedy L[1], Kothari D, Richards RJ.

The mortality rate of toxic megacolon secondary to *C. difficile* colitis is substantial and varies from 38% to 80%[5,13]. Early recognition and aggressive treatment of toxic megacolon associated with *C. difficile* may lead to improved outcomes. Yet, standards for diagnosis and management of this potentially lethal condition are not clearly defined.

http://en.wikipedia.org/wiki/Toxic_megacolon

Toxic Megacolon

****

EMAIL
Ln
No make sauerkraut for 40 years. I do not think it is difficult. How are you feeling today?
Linda
END EMAIL

EMAIL
Claudio is on a rampage because i do not feel good and have Leaky Butt. So i sent him to Cornucopia to buy some Wild Oregano Oil, an antibacterial.
i'll guess you might have called to let me find my phone. Anything else i should have him get?
miso soup good. soba noodles and spinach. yummy
ellen
END EMAIL

```
**************************************************
```

Septicemia

http://www.nlm.nih.gov/medlineplus/ency/article/001355.htm

Septicemia is bacteria in the blood (bacteremia) that often occurs with severe infections.

Alternative Names

Blood poisoning; Bacteremia with sepsis

```
**************************************************
```

EMAIL

Ln

Oh no still leaky butt? It does take time for inflammation to go down.

12-page footnote resource on butt bugs - oh no - when will you get your test back?

Linda

END EMAIL

98.2 F. better than the other day. Under 95 is hypothermia.

https://www.youtube.com/watch?v=81xnvgOlHaY

Interesting Dr. McDougall lecture on the death of Steve Jobs.

EMAIL

LEENDA

Black tea might be what kept it from leaking Christmas Day and yesterday.

today i drank green tea instead. maybe green tea doesn't have tannins. i got progressively worse throughout the day. i am drinking a cup of black tea now.

i have phone in pocket and reading a white paper on clindamycin HCl & *C. difficile*

Damn dentist prescribed the broad-spectrum antibiotic as a preventative and I put it into my mouth. His bad and my bad. Instead the antibiotic caused *Clostridium difficile* infection (CDI), or *Clostridium difficile*-associated diarrhea, (CDAD). Thanks a lot.

The antibiotic Metronidazole (Flagyl) is also used to treat Giardisis and *H. pylori*

COME ON TEA
ellen
END EMAIL

EMAIL
LEENDA
ah dunno
i took the poo in Saturday morning.
hoping for test results tomorrow.
With God, all things are. ~ Margie Pendleton
ellen
END EMAIL

29 DECEMBER, MONDAY

What am I dealing with?
****
http://en.wikipedia.org/wiki/Clostridium_difficile_toxin_B
Toxin B

The role of toxin A and toxin B in *Clostridium difficile* infection
http://www.nature.com/nature/journal/v467/n7316/full/nature09397.html

http://naturalmedicinejournal.net/pdf/nmj_nov09to_clinton.pdf **plant tannins & ulcerative colitis**
"UC has no cure and requires a lifetime of treatment, making accurate diagnosis imperative."

```
*****************************************************
```

No cure. Great! Do I believe this? No.

In general, mankind, since the improvement in cookery, eats twice as much as nature requires. — Benjamin Franklin

FOOD TODAY: Probiotics, black tea, mashed potatoes, carrot juice w/chia seeds, miso soup w/spinach, ginger, garlic and soba noodles, TJs Force Primeval apple/raisin/walnut bars, steamed potatoes with tahini.

EMAIL
SUBJECT: GI Doctor
TO: CW, LEENDA
I am not going to this GI Doctor. Look at their Basic Gluten-Free diet that they recommend:
http://montereygi.com.edit.officite.com/docs/Basic%20Gluten-Free%20Diet.pdf
Preferred foods include **aspartame & MSG**.
Are they idiots????

look at the "Soft Diet" from the Monterey Bay GI Consultants Medical Group; a cast of other doctors:
http://montereygi.com.edit.officite.com/docs/Soft%20Diet.pdf

"Colitis" is not available in their search. What Gastrointestinal medical service does not include "colitis" in their search results?
http://www.montereygi.com/education.html?query=colitis
ellen
END EMAIL

http://en.wikipedia.org/wiki/Diospyros_kaki
Diospyros kaki (Asian persimmon, Japanese persimmon)
The fruit has a high tannin content which makes the immature fruit astringent and bitter. The tannin levels are reduced as the

fruit matures. Persimmons like *Hachiya* must be completely ripened before consumption. When ripe, this fruit comprises thick pulpy jelly encased in a waxy thin skinned shell.
http://en.wikipedia.org/wiki/Persimmon

My Miso Soup tonight:
mushroom broth
mild yellow miso
Braggs Liquid Aminos
ginger
soba noodles
spinach
green onions
yum

30 DECEMBER, TUESDAY *102 pounds*

Leave your drugs in the chemist's pot if you can cure the patient with food.   — Hippocrates

Foods eaten: Probiotics, Kevita, Spicy black tea w/rice milk, banana, TJs Force Primeval apple/raisin/walnut bar, Spicy black bean soup, TJs Green juice and carrot juice, blue corn chips, multi-vitamin, plant-based Chile Relleno, spicy tea w/rice milk, raw persimmon.

Illumina, San Diego:
http://www.illumina.com/
http://www.illumina.com/content/dam/illumina-marketing/documents/products/research_reviews/infectious-

disease-review.pdf

http://www.fda.gov/NewsEvents/Newsroom/PressAnnounce
ments/ucm257024.htm

Clostridium difficile-associated diarrhea (CDAD)
People at risk of developing the bacterial infection include the
elderly, patients in hospitals or nursing homes, and people
taking antibiotics for another infection. The most effective way
to prevent CDAD is thorough handwashing with soap and
warm water.

http://www.aafp.org/afp/2013/0201/p211.html
Fidaxomicin (Dificid) for _Clostridium difficile_ Infection

http://www.anniesremedy.com **Herbal remedies**

http://www.natural-alternative-therapies.com/oil-of-oregano-
uses/ **Oregano**

http://valhallamovement.com/blog/2013/08/22/10-
antibacterial-plants/ **10 antibacterial plants**
Calendula (external), cayenne, garlic, peppermint, rose, St.
John's wort, thyme, cedar, oregano, cinnamon, tea tree.

**Some Common Spices and Plants with Antimicrobial and
Therapeutic Properties**
http://www2.hawaii.edu/~johnb/micro/m140/syllabus/week/
handouts/m140.8.3.html
clove (AB), cinnamon (AB), nutmeg & mace (AB), oregano
(AB), onion (AB), garlic (AB), anise (AB), sassafras, Noni (GI &
liver), wintergreen, ginger (AB).

http://www.researchomatic.com/Antibacterial-Properties-Of-
Plants-124727.html **Antibacterial Properties Of Plants**

http://www.sciencedirect.com/science/article/pii/S138357420 2000078 **Is metronidazole carcinogenic?**

News from the World of Pharmacology
Newly Approved Drugs, New Formulations, New Indications
https://www.lexi.com/individuals/pharmacists/newsletters.jsp?id=july_10
http://www.webmd.com/ibd-crohns-disease/ulcerative-colitis/ss/slideshow-uc-overview ~ **slideshow-uc-overview**

http://www.wired.com/2011/08/killing-beneficial-bacteria/ **gut flora**

31 DECEMBER, WEDNESDAY

Aloe w/no lime, potatoes, herb tea, St. John's Wort w/rice milk, banana, coconut Kevita, carrot juice w/chia seeds.

Dr. Schulze on IBS, colitis:
http://healingtools.tripod.com/thns15.html
****
Botanical Ingredients:
Hawaiian Yellow Ginger Root, Fennel Seed, Peppermint Leaf and Oil
****
https://www.drmcdougall.com/misc/2013stars/starryan.htm
Ryan Schultz, DVM (veterinarian) Cures Himself of Crohn's Disease
"My diet now mostly consists of white sweet potatoes (I don't like the yams as well), brown rice, black beans, spinach, bananas,

oranges, tomatoes, broccoli, peanut butter, and a few nuts."

http://vedgedout.com/why-vegan/

http://www.colitisiq.com
http://www.colitisiq.com/symptoms-of-colitis/#comments
How to Overcome Colitis
ellen, you just completed your payment. $5.00
Your receipt number for this payment is: 2991-8381-1285-5836.
We'll send a confirmation email to espbooks@gmail.com.

No confirmation.   [NOTE: it hasn't arrived yet....]
****
http://www.globalhealingcenter.com/natural-health/liver-
cleanse-foods/ **healthy foods for the liver**

tips for growing medicinal herbs:
http://www.globalhealingcenter.com/organic-herbs
*I just ordered some **Nascent Iodine** from Global Healing
Center. I have taken it before and it's good.*

EMAIL
From: esp [mailto:espbooks@gmail.com]
Sent: Wednesday, December 31, 2014 3:11 PM
To: office@drmcdougall.com
Subject: Antibiotic-induced colitis, *C. diff* infection

Hello Wonderful McDougall Office and HAPPY NEW YEAR'S EVE

I read *The Starch Solution* in August 2012, changed my diet and
have been whole foods plant-based since. Thank you SO much; i
LOVE my diet.

on Dec 19, 2014, diarrhea began without a clue to the cause.

I managed through Christmas Eve.

Christmas Day I went down for the count with abdominal cramps and continued diarrhea.

I tried to figure out why i had diarrhea and traced it back to a tooth extraction and clindamycin HCl Dec. 1, given as a preventative for periodontal procedure. I did not have an infection but the periodontist said the antibiotic was "standard protocol". If I had read the side effects I might not have taken the clindamycin.

I went to a doc in the box and i am waiting for lab test results (especially *Clostridium difficile*). I can eat now and have improved bowel movements but my liver feels tender.

I had never heard of colitis before and from what I am finding on the Internet it looks really nasty with some saying "incurable."

I am not buying into this and intend to get well. I have searched the drmcdougall.com website for colitis but found only one reference. I am already animal-free, dairy-free, sugar-free, organic, chemical-free, oil-free, etc.

What plant-based guidance might you offer?

I have been taking probiotics, aloe, many antibacterial herbs, potatoes, and I LOVE the Miso Soup recipe in *The Starch Solution* to which I have added spinach, mushroom broth, ginger and soba noodles.

The beautiful SILVER LINING in this, so far, is that I now see food as medicine. I've been eating well, but my focus and perspective has shifted through this.

I am a 62-year-old female, mother, grandmother, author and backpacker (I took McDougall cups-of-soups backpacking LONG before I knew about plant-based cuz they were the best). Colitis really sucks.

It is my intention to beat this. If I do, maybe I could become a Star McDougaller????

thank you for your time and attention.

enJOY

Ellen Pendleton

END EMAIL

To: Quest Diagnostics
HAPPY NEW YEAR
I had blood tests on Dec. 26 and stool samples on Dec. 27 checking for *C. difficile*. I am eager to get the lab results to determine if i have been infectious. I cooked Christmas Eve Dinner and would like to know.

Plus, I am still in bed feeling weak, awaiting test results to decide what to do.
please call
Ellen Pendleton
END EMAIL

http://www.ncbi.nlm.nih.gov/pmc/articles/PMC4146460
testing for Toxin A & B

http://www.globalhealingcenter.com/benefits-of/grapefruit-seed-extract **~ Grapefruit-seed-extract**

http://www.bellaonline.com/articles/art22343.asp
Treating *C-Difficile* with Alternative Medicine

http://www.cdc.gov/HAI/organisms/cdiff/Cdiff-current-strain.html
Information about the Current Strain of *Clostridium difficile*

http://www.naturalnews.com/039826_c_diff_superbug_infections.html
***Clostridium difficile* antibiotic-resistant infections rapidly spreading in hospitals worldwide**

http://www.naturalnews.com/041713_garlic_antibiotics_super bugs.html
As antibiotics continue to fail, use garlic instead to kill MRSA and superbugs

McDougall colitis

Lactobacillus plantarum ~ probiotic

**http://www.nealhendrickson.com/mcdougall/021100pucha
ined.htm** ~ Old McDougall article

Diet for the Treatment of Chronic Colitis

Obviously, the contents of the bowel must have a determining effect upon its health. Therefore, logic dictates that a person wishing to keep his/her bowels healthy should put good foods in them. Whether it is heart disease, cancer, obesity or diabetes that is being discussed, the diet that is recommended is a diet high in complex carbohydrates and low in animal foods and fats – in other words a plant-based diet. There should be no surprise that the same diet is "bowel-healthy" too.

I believe the best diet for preventing and treating all forms of colitis is based upon starches with the addition of fruits and vegetables. This diet is also devoid of all free fats (all vegetable oils) and all animal products. If this fails to resolve the problems then the next step is to eliminate wheat products. Finally, the elimination diet should be tried to search out any offending foods. With this approach I have seen most people with colitis improve and many cured of their conditions – including those with the more serious forms of IBD. There is no reason not to believe this and try a healthy diet for a period of time (say 4 months). There are no added costs and no side effects from this approach and there is a real possibility of excellent health being the result.

http://www.nealhendrickson.com/mcdougall/2004nl/041100p
ufavorite5.htm

Ulcerative Colitis Relapses with Meat and Beef
Influence of dietary factors on the clinical course of ulcerative colitis: a prospective cohort study by Sarah L. Jowett in the October 2004 issue of the journal *Gut* found patients with ulcerative colitis had more frequent relapses when they consumed meat, especially red and processed meat, and eggs.[1] The investigators felt the risk of relapse, and thus the activity, was from the sulfur compounds found in these animal foods. Alcoholic beverages, many of which contain sulfur compounds, were also associated with risk of relapse.

Comment: Ulcerative colitis is a disease that causes inflammation and sores, called ulcers, in the lining of primarily the large intestine. The inflammation occurs most commonly in the rectum and lower part of the colon, but it may affect the entire colon. This painful inflammatory bowel disease (IBD) can be debilitating (diarrhea and stomach pains), and even fatal.

To begin to understand the cause of this disease, you must know that ulcerative colitis is found only in parts of the world where people follow the Western diet, high in meat and dairy foods. This is an autoimmune disease, where the immune system attacks the body (in this case, the bowel primarily).

The course of ulcerative colitis is characterized by frequent exacerbations (relapses). Previous studies have found a high intake of dairy products, and a low intake of dietary fiber, are associated with relapses. Patients with ulcerative colitis also have higher concentrations of sulfur in their intestines and the course of the disease correlates with that amount.[2] Sulfur appears to be toxic to the intestine. So, where does all this sulfur come from?

The amount of sulfur in the intestine is increased by consuming animal products, which are inherently high in sulfur-containing amino acids, like methionine and cysteine.

Sulfur-Containing Amino Acids
- Beef provides 4 times more than pinto beans
- Eggs have 4 times more than corn
- Cheddar cheese has 5 times more than white potatoes
- Chicken provides 7 times more than rice
- Tuna provides 12 times more than sweet potatoes

Dramatic improvement in patients with ulcerative colitis has been reported with a change to a diet low in sulfur-containing amino acids.[2] My experience has been that people with ulcerative colitis, and a similar condition called Crohn's disease, respond quickly and dramatically with a change to the diet we recommend (starch-based with the addition of fruits and vegetables). This is a diet which is inherently low in sulfur compounds because the foods we recommend contain no animal-derived products.

1) Jowett SL, Seal CJ, Pearce MS, Phillips E, Gregory W, Barton JR, Welfare MR. Influence of dietary factors on the clinical course of ulcerative colitis: a prospective cohort study. *Gut.* 2004 Oct;53(10):1479-84.

2) Roediger WE. Decreased sulphur aminoacid intake in ulcerative colitis. *Lancet.* 1998 May 23;351(9115):1555.

https://www.drmcdougall.com/misc/2005nl/august/050800pro.htm ~ **probiotics McDougall**

Bifidobacterium
<u>Ulcerative Colitis:</u>
Escherichia coli, Nissle strain (1917)
BIFICO (3 *Bifidobacteria* species)
Saccharomyces boulardii
VLS 3 brand (*Lactobacillus and Bifidobacteria*)

http://www.Kevita.com
Kevita Blueberry Cherry and Mango Coconut
Bacillus coagulans GBI-30 6086
L. rhamnosus
L. paracasei
L. plantarum

http://www.ncbi.nlm.nih.gov/pmc/articles/PMC3484022/
Bacillus coagulans GBI-30, 6086 limits the recurrence of Clostridium difficile-Induced colitis following vancomycin withdrawal in mice

http://www.vsl3.com
VSL#3 high-potency probiotic medical food contains 8 different strains of live lactic acid bacteria that were specially selected to produce an optimal synergistic composition of bacteria. The 8 strains are:

- *Bifidobacterium breve*
- *Bifidobacterium longum*
- *Bifidobacterium infantis*
- *Lactobacillus acidophilus*
- *Lactobacillus plantarum*

- *Lactobacillus paracasei*
- *Lactobacillus bulgaricus*
- *Streptococcus thermophilus*

VSL#3 products may contain trace amounts of lactose [0.1g per 100g] and dehydrated skim milk or milk protein (casein and beta-lacto globulin of less than 2mg/Kg).

No casein for me. [See: The China Study]

https://www.utopiasilver.com/testimonials/colitis/
Colloidal Silver
****

TRIBE.NET BLOG
http://tribes.tribe.net/herbalmedicine/thread/546f432d-94ad-4373-a07f-87b72798b151 ~ **Forum, blog, tribes:**
Jarrow *Saccharomyces boulardii*
Apple Cider Vinegar - two Tbs. twice daily in water (with honey) is an oldie but goodie

EM,

I am really beginning to understand the importance of bacterial communication. Apparently in this situation, Bacteria A in some fashion, spoken in basic terms, 'eats' Bacteria B's poop. When bacteria A is killed off via antibiotics, there begins an unbalance in the system. It's not that C-diff is 'bad', guess it's simply that the C-Diff's excrement is not being taken care of and ends up building up to toxic levels.

The part that confuses me the most is that prior to my having an overpopulation of *C. diff*, I haven't been on antibiotics in over 3-4 years. So that is not the culprit behind my 'infestation' or whatever it is.

I finished the Vanco, and on the 7-8th day of the 10 day

prescription, the symptoms of this subsided. It was one of the worst things I've ever gone through. When there wasn't food to leave my body I just bled when I went to the bathroom.. a lot.

My GI's NP is awesome and listens wayyyy more than my GI, so I usually just try to talk to her. She wrote me a script for VSL-3 but asked me not to take it b4 I was done with the Vanco as they don't yet know how one will effect the efficacy of the other. So I waited and started taking it after the script of Vanco. I take 4 pills a day, 2 morn / 2 night. Plus I am drinking Lifeway's Organic, Plain Kefir Daily. I'm eating primarily what I want, although lately I've noticed an increased intolerance to citrus via WICKED Canker Sores on my tongue and insides of my cheeks. I can't speak when I get them and swallowing is difficult because my tongue swells up where the sore is. This is a new thing now and I feel like I just can't catch a damn break. So any info about the root cause of Canker Sores would be beneficial as well.

The nurse shared with me that eating too many Organic Foods can lead to a C-Diff infection because there are many foods that are high in natural antibiotics such as mushrooms. I had no idea. I'm beginning to wonder if there is any way for me to heal and be healthy again. I just kind of feel like a shell of the person I was.

ps... i wish there weren't so many deleted posts. i never got a chance to read them and as this was my thread, i am interested in what everyone has to say regardless of how polite or impolite it is. not trying to be rude, just honest. i was bummed to see there were posts that i could not have the opportunity to read before they were removed.

BLOG CONTINTUES:

Re: Virulent Bacteria "C-Diff"

Mon, June 22, 2009 - 7:46 AM

"The nurse shared with me that eating too many Organic Foods can lead to a *C-Diff* infection because there are many foods that are high in natural antibiotics such as mushrooms. I had no idea. I'm beginning to wonder if there is any way for me to heal and be healthy again. I just kind of feel like a shell of the person I was."

I think on that particular note that the nurse had no idea of what she was talking about. A better way to make her point would have been something like 'don't eat certain foods without researching them, such as some mushrooms' - organic shouldn't have something to do with it. I'd guess that they might see people for this condition, who happen to eat organic because they've been sick for a few years and have changed their diet to try to fix the digestive system problem, not that they have a digestive system problem because of organic foods.

Contagious????

When a bacterium comes in contact with an unfavourable environment, it turns into a spore to survive. The bacterium membrane will form into a hard shell protecting the bacterium's DNA inside. Once that spore comes in contact with a favourable environment, the spore becomes active again, so the hard shell cracks and the DNA becomes active the bacteriums membrane is back, and it begins to replicate every 20 minutes or so. This spore form *C.diff* is highly resistant to heat and would probably pass through the stomach acid and the alkaline enzymes of the small intestine processes, finally finding it's way into the neutral colon where it will go boom.
You would find these spores probably in and around the toilet area, someone would just put their hand on the handle of the door, have something to eat or drink later, and the bacterium found its way in, it's that easy.
You're more at risk to *C.diff* if your immune is suppressed in any way, be that from age, other medical conditions, certain medications, even pregnancy.

There would be different strains of *C.diff* just like there's different strains of Golden staph, unfortunately you may have picked up a more virulent strain in the hospital. Vanc is the only effective antibiotic left that i know of, on top of that even if you have a correct pH balance with all the correct flora bacteria in your colon, *C. diff* will still go unchecked as it uses different nutrients to replicate to that of beneficial bacteria.

Not all is lost being that you just had a baby, your immune system would have been struggling, and this would of given the upper hand to the *C.diff,* now that you're hopefully on to recovery, once your immune systems back up to it's full potential you would have a better chance of fighting the bacteria off, more than likely with the help of vanc.

Eating the right foods to improve your immune system may help too, like vitamin and enzyme rich foods. I'm guessing the charcoal would help absorb the toxins that *C. diff* gives off in the colon. I don't like antibiotics myself but everything has its place, using vanc to get rid of or cutting the numbers of *C. diff* down would definitely help and give your immune system a better chance to catch up.

I hope this helped, and I hope you get better soon.

- Craig

END BLOG

****

frankincense *(Boswellia serrata)* The *Physicians Desk Reference for Herbal Medicines* recommends taking a gum resin preparation of 350mg of frankincense three times a day for 6 weeks.

slippery elm

The Physicians Desk Reference for Medicinal Herbs
http://academic.uprm.edu/dpesante/docs-apicultura/pdr%20para%20la%20medicina%20herbal.pdf
for irritable bowel syndrome: Asa Foetida (also good for liver disorders), peppermint, psyllium, and psyllium seed

fenugreek, rice.

Clostridium difficile in adults: Treatment
http://www.uptodate.com/contents/clostridium-difficile-in-adults-treatment?source=see_link

Fecal Transplant:
http://www.uptodate.com/contents/fecal-microbiota-transplantation-in-the-treatment-of-recurrent-clostridium-difficile-infection?source=related_link)

http://www.uptodate.com/contents/clostridium-difficile-and-probiotics?source=see_link) [~ *Great list of resources!*]
http://www.uptodate.com/contents/clostridium-difficile-and-probiotics?source=see_link

MECHANISMS OF PROBIOTICS
Both *lactobacilli* [14] and *S. boulardii* [15] have been shown to suppress the growth of *C. difficile* in hamsters.

Saccharomyces boulardii
http://en.wikipedia.org/wiki/Saccharomyces_boulardii
Saccharomyces boulardii is a tropical strain of **yeast** first isolated from **lychee** and **mangosteen** fruit in 1923 by French scientist Henri Boulard.
****

I buy some:

Jarrow *Saccharomyces boulardii,* 5 billion **and take two.**
http://www.jarrow.com/product/265/Saccharomyces_Boulardii_MOS

Kevita Blueberry Cherry ~ *mangosteen in ingredients*
Bacillus coagulans GBI-30 6086
L. rhamnosus
L. paracasei
L. plantarum

https://www.drmcdougall.com/misc/2005nl/august/050800pr

https://www.youtube.com/watch?v=h0CQrL5nzwo
War on Health - Gary Null's documentary exposing the FDA

~ Happy New Year!!! ~

1 January 2015, Thursday

The art of healing comes from nature, not from the physician. Therefore the physician must start from nature, with an open mind.
— Philipus Aureolus Paracelsus

Aloe, probiotic, milk thistle, glutathione, oregano, kelp, sweetie potatoes (added pumpkin pie spices), rice milk, more milk thistle, TJs organic hummus, avocado, Quinoa pasta: fresh tomatoes, spinach, olives (Kalamata, green and black), onions, garlic, turmeric, oregano, basil, fennel seeds, salt, white pepper, frozen artichoke hearts.

2 January, Friday
My Beloved

Reality is that which when you stop believing in it ... doesn't go away.
— Philip K. Dick

Aloe, rice milk, apple, Kevita, banana, brown rice, black

bean soup, raw garlic, charcoal, colloidal silver, ginger tea, potatoes, kelp, potassium iodide, walnuts, electrolytes.

EMAIL
OK, Children and Tom.
The shit has hit the fan.

THE BAD NEWS IS:

The lab test detected *Toxigenic Clostridium difficile* and i may have have been infectious all of the Christmas season and may still be. It's a hygiene issue. Alcohol-based hand sanitizers don't work; soap and water hand-washing works. Hopefully I did not infect any of you with Christmas dinner and meal preparations. Yes, this sucks and I am so sorry. I did not know I was infectious. If you or anyone close to you get ANY diarrhea call me or go to a doctor immediately and get tested for *C. difficile.* The diarrhea symptom can take a while to show up. It took two weeks to show up for me and it can sometimes take months. DO NOT TAKE ANTIDIARRHEAL MEDICATIONS, such as Imodium.

THE GOOD NEWS:
I intend to wrestle this and win.
I just got home from Doc in the Box and will research healing options. Thank goodness for the Internet.

http://en.wikipedia.org/wiki/Clostridium_difficile_colitis

Garlic, probiotics, grapefruit seed extract, aloe, oil of oregano, charcoal, turmeric, many healthy options are available and i am on it. I welcome input.

So up your probiotics. (I'll mail some to you as soon as I can.) Eat some raw garlic, kimchi, sauerkraut, kefir, yogurt, miso and Blueberry Cherry Kevita Sparkling Probiotic drink (w/mangosteen).

And don't take antibiotics as a preventative before oral surgery, damn it. I took a broad-spectrum antibiotic, clindamycin HCl. I was healthy, went to the dentist and now i have antibiotic-induced pseudomembranous colitis. I do not want any of you to get this!!!!

Stay well. Be aware. Live Large. Think. Intuit. Dance. Celebrate.
LOVE and TRUST. call if you want. i am not going anywhere.
LOVE to you
~ yoMama

No replies of diarrhea.

*Kevita Blueberry Cherry has the probiotic GBI-30 6086
and is getting rave reviews for dealing with C. difficile:*
http://www.ncbi.nlm.nih.gov/pmc/articles/PMC3484022/
*I've been drinking one a day since Christmas, taking
another Lactobacilli from CVS and eating miso soup. I
actually bought some sauerkraut today from Trader Joe's.
I've never tasted sauerkraut before. This should be
interesting.*

3 JANUARY, SATURDAY *100 POUNDS*

*Colloidal silver, glutamine, grapefruit seed extract, oil of
oregano, aloe, B12, peppermint oil, milk thistle,
Blueberry Cherry Kevita, amaranth (w/flaxseed meal, 1/2
banana, cinnamon), Medicinal Indian Hummus, avocado,
TJs raw sauerkraut w/Persian pickles (just a taste), carrot
juice w/psyllium fiber, miso soup (soba noodles, ginger,
garlic, spinach, asparagus, green onions), colloidal silver.*

EMAIL
Hi Mom
I'd recommend at least 50 billion strain probiotic from the cold
section in whatever health food store you want to go to. My Dr
recommended you get the most strains possible when you're using

them restoratively. Also, take a really good quality enzyme before each meal.
Also, if you're not eating oil, where are you getting your omega 3's?
Love u. Sunshine
END EMAIL

Sunshine is my daughter. We had Christmas Eve dinner at her house.

EMAIL
Hi Sweetheart
Oh you are brilliant and an excellent resource. Thank you.

Okay. I'll get the 50 billion. Kevita has 4 billion. The CVS Pearls have 15 billion. Thank you for your help here. *Merci.*

What enzyme? I don't think that i have any.

I am eating fresh fruit (apples, bananas) and lightly steamed veggies, (asparagus, cauliflower, spinach), raw garlic and lots of miso soup. I am mono eating, except the miso soup. Potatoes, brown rice, black bean soup, nutritional yeast rules! I have to gain weight so i am going to try some tofu today and maybe an avocado. I weighed in today at 100.0 pounds.

I'll look into omega 3's. I'm not knowledgeable about this. Here's my uneducated sense: Don't we need the omega 3's to balance out the ratio of omega 6? And omega 6 comes from animals? And if i don't eat animals that have omega 6 then i don't need omega 3 supplements to balance?

I know flaxseeds have a lot of omega 3s so i will work flaxseed meal into my diet. 1800 mg in 2 Tbls. I'll try amaranth too.

Thank you Dahlin'. More to learn. I spent yesterday in bed on my laptop and woke up with a sore shoulder this morning. Bonnie Prudden pressure, comfrey lotion and i feel good to go.

and no coffee. The organic green bean oven-roasted coffee days were good and now they are over.

I welcome your input, feedback, advice, recommendations, hints, clues, and love.

~ yoMama

Mom
These are the enzymes I have:
Pharmaca Chewable Papaya Enzymes
Rainbow Light Advanced Enzyme System
Natural Factors Multi Enzyme High Potency
  Vegetarian Formula
SS

nice.
i used to take enzymes.
thank you, this helps.

i am gonna eat an avocado.

Then I'm gonna make some Medicinal Indian Hummus with tahini, golden raisins, extra turmeric, extra raw garlic and no oil. YUMMY

For dinner i'll make some miso soup with soba noodles. my appetite has returned.

Could you see the moon set the last two nights? Unbelievable. RedOrange on the horizon. Amazing.

~ yoMama

4 JANUARY, SUNDAY

Black tea, potato, Medicinal Indian Hummus, miso soup, cooked apples, raw persimmon, herbs, supplements, Kevita, carrot juice w/psyllium fiber, ABCALM® (freeze-dried calcium, magnesium), colloidal silver.

http://www.ncbi.nlm.nih.gov/pmc/articles/PMC522321/
Performance of the TechLab *C. DIFF* CHEK-60 Enzyme Immunoassay (EIA) in Combination with the *C. difficile* Tox A/B II EIA Kit, the Triage *C. difficile* Panel Immunoassay, and a Cytotoxin Assay for Diagnosis of *Clostridium difficile*-Associated Diarrhea

http://www.ncbi.nlm.nih.gov/pmc/articles/PMC105000/
Identification of Toxin A-Negative, Toxin B-Positive *Clostridium difficile* by PCR

http://jmm.sgmjournals.org/content/53/2/167.full
Clostridium difficile colonization in healthy adults: transient colonization and correlation with enterococcal colonization

Effect of tea phenolics and their aromatic fecal bacterial metabolites on intestinal microbiota
http://www.sciencedirect.com/science/article/pii/S0923250806001525

****
http://www.ncbi.nlm.nih.gov/pmc/articles/PMC86532/
Pseudomembranous Colitis Caused by a Toxin $A^- B^+$ Strain of *Clostridium difficile* ~ includes case studies.

REFERENCES
1. al-Barrak A, Embil J, Dyck B, Olekson K, Nicoll D, Alfa M, Kabani A. **An outbreak of toxin A negative, toxin B positive**

Clostridium difficile-associated diarrhea in a Canadian tertiary-care hospital. Can Commun Dis Rep. 1999;25:65–69. [PubMed]

2. Bongaerts G P A, Lyerly D M. **Role of bacterial metabolism and physiology in the pathogenesis of** *Clostridium difficile* **disease.** Microb Pathog. 1997;2:253–256. [PubMed]

3. Brazier J S. **The diagnosis of** *Clostridium difficile*-**associated disease.** J Antimicrob Ther. 1998;41(Suppl. C):29–40. [PubMed]

4. Kato H, Kato N, Katow S, Maegawa T, Nakamura S, Lyerly D M. **Deletions in the repeating sequences of the toxin A gene of toxin A-negative, toxin B-positive** *Clostridium difficile* **strains.** FEMS Microbiol Lett. 1999;175:197–203. [PubMed]

5. Kato H, Kato N, Watanabe K, Iwai N, Nakamura H, Yamamoto T, Suzuki K, Kim S-M, Chong Y, Wasito E B. **Identification of a toxin A-negative, toxin B-positive** *Clostridium difficile* by PCR. J Clin Microbiol. 1998;36:2178–2182. [PMC free article] [PubMed]

6. Knoop F C, Owens M, Crocker I C. *Clostridium difficile*: **clinical disease and diagnosis.** Clin Microbiol Rev. 1993;6:251–265. [PMC free article] [PubMed]

7. Lyerly D M, Barroso L A, Wilkins T D, Depitre C, Corthier G. **Characterization of a toxin A-negative, toxin B-positive strain of** *Clostridium difficile.* Infect Immun. 1992;60:4633–4639. [PMC free article] [PubMed]

8. Lyerly D M, Krivan H C, Wilkins T D. *Clostridium difficile*: **its disease and toxins.** Clin Microbiol Rev. 1988;1:1–18. [PMC free article] [PubMed]

9. Lyerly D M, Neville L M, Evans D T, Fill J, Allen S, Greene W, Sautter R, Hnatuck P, Torpey D J, Schwalbe R. **Multicenter evaluation of the** *Clostridium difficile* **TOX A/B Test.** J Clin Microbiol. 1998;36:184–190. [PMC free article] [PubMed]

10. Surawicz C M, McFarland L V. **Pseudomembranous colitis: causes and cures.** Digestion. 1999;60:91–100. [PubMed]

****

http://cmr.asm.org/content/18/2/247.full

Clostridium difficile Toxins: Mechanism of Action and Role in Disease
****
http://www.questdiagnostics.com/testcenter/TestDetail.action?ntc=91664 ~ **Toxin/GDH W/R**

http://www.easy-immune-health.com/blood-test-abbreviations.html ~ **blood test abbreviations**

~ PHAGE, PROBIOTICS AND PREBIOTICS ~

5 JANUARY, MONDAY *102 pounds*

Red grapefruit juice, avocado, walnuts, Kevita, aloe, herbs, supplements, milk thistle, peppermint, B12, grapefruit seed extract, oregano, fenugreek, vegan electrolytes, kelp, potassium iodide, small piece of Trader Joe's Force Primeval Bars - raisin/walnut/apple bars, small piece of rice cake, ginger tea, Persian dal w/roasted butternut squash, potato, carrot juice.

Evergreen Phage Lab:
http://blogs.evergreen.edu/phage/

Evergreen YouTube Channel:
https://www.youtube.com/channel/UC-JKKD48WjA3rbC-oeqWjBg

http://en.wikipedia.org/wiki/Phage_therapy
As has been known for at least thirty years, mycobacteria such as *Mycobacterium tuberculosis* have specific bacteriophages. No lytic phage has yet been discovered for *Clostridium difficile*, which is responsible for many nosocomial diseases, but some *temperate phages* (integrated in the genome) are known for this species, which opens encouraging avenues.

http://www.ncbi.nlm.nih.gov/pmc/articles/PMC2786741/
Thus, it appears that *C. difficile* strains often harbor temperate phage(s) as part of their genetic makeup. No direct evidence of lysogenic conversion of a nontoxinogenic *C. difficile* strain to toxin production was shown. However, preliminary results showed that toxin A and/or toxin B production is modified in a toxigenic *C. difficile* lysogen. In our lab we have successfully used a *C. difficile* phage for treating *C. difficile*-associated disease in hamster models. Later, we characterized and presented the first complete *C. difficile* phage genome. During these studies it was found that ΦCD119 could modulate toxin production in its *C. difficile* host strains.

http://www.ncbi.nlm.nih.gov/pmc/articles/PMC1428422/
phage

Nucleotide sequence accession number.
The genome from phage ΦCD119 was deposited in GenBank under accession number AY855346.

http://www.ncbi.nlm.nih.gov/genome/5740 ~ **phage CD119**

http://www.phageinternational.com/ **Phage International**

http://www.phagetherapy.com/imc/IMCGServlet?command=static_home ~ **NovoMed Georgia**

http://www.phageinternational.com/press.htm ~ **press**

Environmental Response and Autoregulation of
Clostridium difficile TxeR, a Sigma Factor for Toxin Gene
Expression
http://www.ncbi.nlm.nih.gov/pmc/articles/PMC135396/

Effect of arginine on toxin production by *Clostridium
difficile* in defined medium. Walnuts
http://www.ncbi.nlm.nih.gov/pubmed/9310936

http://www.google.com/patents/US20120177608
phage patent

Casey Harlington ~ investor for Georgia Research Institute

http://en.wikipedia.org/wiki/Giorgi_Eliava_Institute

Eliava Institute in Tbilisi, Georgia
http://www.eliava-institute.org/?rid=8&pg=2

http://www.ncbi.nlm.nih.gov/pubmed/2258909
**12th C. L. Oakley lecture. Pathogenesis of *Clostridium
difficile* infection of the gut.**

http://www.phagetherapycenter.com/pii/PatientServlet?
command=static_ptwhitepapers&language=0
Phage Therapy Center ~ White Papers and News Articles

BBC Video on Bacteriophage ~ 59 minutes
https://www.phagetherapycenter.com/virusthatcures.mp4
This video has amazing information! I LOVE PHAGE! They
look like little aliens. This video helps to explain SO much!

http://www.bbc.com/news/health-21799534
Eliava Institute in Tbilisi, Georgia

https://www.youtube.com/watch?v=FEjNMlNM3l8#t=60
Part III
Dr. Alan MacDonald- Pathologist Lyme Disease Expert

Rise of Superbugs ~ video
http://www.dailymotion.com/video/xvxd9k_rise-of-the-superbugs_news?start=456

SuperInfection
http://en.wikipedia.org/wiki/Superinfection
****
EMAIL
From: Sharon@drmcdougall.com
Date: Mon, Jan 5, 2015 at 2:18 PM
Subject: RE: Antibiotic-induced colitis, *C. diff* infection
To: esp <espbooks@gmail.com>
Ellen
Sounds like you are doing everything that you can do right now. I, too, would suspect that the medication is what brought on your colitis. Just keep eating the way you have been eating and it should resolve itself. Although it will probably take longer than you would hope. Taking the probiotics is probably a good idea to help regain some colon bacteria.
END EMAIL

EMAIL
From: <espbooks@gmail.com>
Date: Mon, Jan 5, 2015 at 10:02 PM
Subject: Re: Antibiotic-induced colitis, *C. diff* infection
To: Sharon

Hi Sharon

Thank you so for your reply.

I got the lab results on Friday which detected Toxigenic *C. difficile*. Doc in the Box prescribed Flagyl but i told them i wouldn't take it. "Why?" she asked. "Because it is a potential carcinogen banned in

59

the European Union and in the USA for use in animals." Then she told me very out loud in front of the entire waiting room full, "If you don't take it the doctor says that you will end up in the hospital from dehydration." WOW.

I am not taking them.

I am actually feeling pretty good and my BMs are very improved. They're not stellar yet but moving that direction (excuse the pun).
I have gained three pounds back weighing in this morning at 103.
YIPPEEE SKIIPPPEEE

I LOVE my diet.

In my Internet research today i came upon phage therapy and watched a BBC video about an institute in Georgia, near Russia, dedicated to this. It noted finding four strains of *C. difficile* but no phage yet. It's fascinating and a possible way out of the antibiotic resistant world.

I am eating raw garlic, drinking antibacterial herb teas, aloe, keeping on my diet, drinking black and green tea occasionally and eager to know wellness again.

Any insight, tips, clues, advice, recommendations regarding *C. difficile* and precautions for my future?

Thank you SO much for being

enJOY
Ellen Pendleton

PS ~ I am eager to go out to play
END EMAIL

6 JANUARY, TUESDAY

Nobody seems more obsessed by diet than our anti-materialistic, otherworldly, New Age spiritual types. But if the material world is

merely illusion, an honest guru should be as content with Budweiser and bratwurst as with raw carrot juice, tofu and seaweed slime.
— Edward Abbey

Aloe, probiotics, herbs, supplements, colloidal silver, two cups Spicy Chai black tea w/stevia & almond milk, avocado, banana, potato w/nutritional yeast & almond meal, Medicinal Indian Hummus, (I call it *medicinal* because I add extra raw garlic and turmeric), canned artichoke hearts in water, steamed asparagus, brown rice and black bean soup, applesauce, ...

EMAIL
From: Scout
Date: Tue, Jan 6, 2015 at 8:53 AM
Subject: RE: Whales
To: esp <espbooks@gmail.com>

Sat north of Soberanes yesterday. It was gorgeous. The whales are so beautiful. Can you get out of bed yet? I'd come to see you but afraid I might get you sick.
END EMAIL

EMAIL
From: <espbooks@gmail.com>
Date: Tue, Jan 6, 2015 at 9:02 AM
Subject: RE: Whales
To: Scout
Nope
Not outta bed.
Nope, don't bring any sickness
What do you have?
Sinus issues?
Raw garlic rules!

Bacteria, viruses and phage are very interesting!
I watched a BBC video yesterday about this. Wow.

Lemme go weigh in for the day.

101.8 pounds
i thought i would weigh more today.
I'll eat another avocado and more walnuts.

Love to you.
ellen
END EMAIL

EMAIL
From: Sharon
Date: Tue, Jan 6, 2015 at 4:06 PM
Subject: RE: Antibiotic-induced colitis, *C. diff* infection
To: espbooks@gmail.com
Ellen
I have no further insight except for you to keep on with what you
are doing. It sounds like you are getting some positive results and i
would expect these to continue as long as you continue to eat this
way. Beware of "falling off the wagon" though. It's easy to get back
into trouble quickly.
END EMAIL

EMAIL
From: <espbooks@gmail.com>
Date: Tue, Jan 6, 2015 at 4:39 PM
Subject: Re: Antibiotic-induced colitis, *C. diff* infection
To: Sharon

Thank you Sharon.

This was such a scare that i don't see "falling off the wagon".

I've been on the McDougall diet over two years and i can list each
wagon falling:
Organic coconut oil, TheLaughingGiraffe.com nuggets about six
months ago.

Had some Brie about a year ago.
Tried a nibble of Bleu Cheese about six months ago and, i swear my guts locked up. How is that possible?

and I went through a vegan cheesecake recipe finding phase that used coconut oil. Yum.

I am on the diet and i LOVE it. Friends and family give me such a hard time because i am very strict with food. I also have MSG allergy and huge sensitivities to chemicals, food additives and ingredients that i cannot pronounce.

With the clindamycin HCl, *C. difficile* and colitis i am not a happy camper with the thought that this could follow me the rest of my life. The only "falling off the wagon" i did, i guess, was taking the preventative antibiotic. It slipped through my awareness and the pain of the dental work. That was my lesson. I will not take antibiotics again as a preventative and always READ THE INSERT.

Thank you, Sharon.
I weighed in this morning at 101.8 so i am eating nuts and avocados trying to gain some weight back.

I hope no one else gets the rude awakening like i did. I'm old, 62. But if this happened to a young one they might have to live with colitis or the threat of it their entire life. That would be sad.

Aloe, raw garlic and oregano rule!!!!!

Thank you for all that you do and for this communication. It helps. I am still bedridden so you've helped to brighten my day. Thank you.

ellen
END EMAIL

7 JANUARY, WEDNESDAY

Part of the secret of success in life is to eat what you like and let the food fight it out inside. — Mark Twain

Probiotics, herbs, supplements, water, colloidal silver, amaranth w/banana walnuts and pumpkin pie spice, apple, rice milk w/saffron, sauerkraut, Persian dal w/butternut squash, aloe, VSL#3 - 2 tabs, ...

http://campother.blogspot.com/2011/04/phage-therapy-and-borrelia-burgdorferi.html *Lyme Borrelias*
Phage Therapy and *Borrelia burgdorferi* (bacteria)

http://www.phagetherapy.com/imc/IMCGServlet?command=static_home
NovoMed, another phage center in Georgia.

http://www.phagetherapy.com/imc/IMCGServlet?command=chronicinfections&secnavpos=3&language=0
NovoMed Chronic and Difficult to Treat Infections

http://pandorareport.org/tag/c-difficile/
The Pandora Report which leads to:
https://www2.le.ac.uk/offices/press/press-releases/2013/october/bacteria-eating-viruses-2018magic-bullets-in-the-war-on-superbugs2019 ~ **University of Leicester, phage Dr. Clokie.** *She claims to have found phage for CDIFF*
https://soundcloud.com/university-of-leicester/martha-clokie-superbugs ~ **podcast**

http://www.leicestermercury.co.uk/Leicester-university-scientists-make-hospital/story-19941276-detail/story.html
A specialist team of scientists from the University of Leicester has isolated viruses that eat bacteria — called phages — to specifically target the highly infectious hospital superbug *Clostridium difficile* (*C. diff*).
Dropbox photos to copy and podcast link:

https://www.dropbox.com/sh/o4rzbs0s156lt06/LwbNj1Vfcc

This is the most exciting thing that I've read!!!
I email: er134@mail.cfs.le.ac.uk but get an autoresponse that Dr. Clokie is out of town at a phage conference. I'll try again.
****
http://jmm.sgmjournals.org/content/54/2/101.full
Alternative treatments for *Clostridium difficile* disease: what really works?

http://www.ncbi.nlm.nih.gov/pubmed/22318930
Fidaxomicin for the treatment of *Clostridium difficile* infections

http://www.ampliphibio.com/news.html
AmpliPhi Biosciences Corporation ~ USA

http://www.dificid.com/understanding/index.php
fidaxomicin or Dificid
http://www.dificid.com/downloads/Dificid_PI.pdf

http://www.ampliphibio.com/news.html
phage therapy *C. difficile* AmpliPhi Biosciences

photos & podcast
https://www.dropbox.com/sh/o4rzbs0s156lt06/LwbNj1Vfcc

http://en.wikipedia.org/wiki/Ethylenediaminetetraacetic_acid
EDTA

http://www.germaware.com/hot-topics/1-latest-news/115-c-diff-superbug.html ~ **GermAware.com**
this blog is scary with many entries.

I am writing a comment on the above blog:

COMMENT: I just went through the broad-spectrum antibiotic clindamycin HCl as a infection preventative measure for a dental procedure. Three weeks later diarrhea, starting with no apparent cause, turned into mucous balls. Went to bed Christmas day and have been here since. Black tea stopped the diarrhea. Started probiotics. Lab results detected TOXIGENIC C. DIFFICILE.

I refused Flagyl. Metronidazole/Flagyl is a potential carcinogen banned in the European Union and the USA for use on animals. I am not taking it. I eat a plant-based diet with no oil, following the Dr. Caldwell Esselstyn and Dr. John McDougall diet. My appetite returned but I am not gaining back weight yet. I weighed in at 102 this morning, stopped the black tea yesterday and had an almost normal BM today. I wonder where all the food is going. No more gut wrenching abdominal cramps, no more diarrhea but I am still weak and afraid to leave the house/toilet. How contagious am I??? I cooked Christmas Eve dinner for my grown children and grandchildren. I told all of them to up their probiotics and if they have any diarrhea take it seriously. What can I do? My body feels much, much improved but after reading all of these blog entries I am feeling rather frightened; fearing relapse; fearing that I may have given C. difficile to my family; fearing that the C. difficile will wreak havoc in everyone's life.

I have been learning about phage therapy and noticed that Bacteriophage for *CDIFF* may have been discovered last October at the University of Leicester. Can anyone tell me how long it might take between discovery of a phage and its availability for public consumption?

May we all be well, happy and healthy. namaste.
END COMMENT
****
GermAware.com WOULDN'T ADD MY COMMENT w/out registration and login. Oh well. I am spent.

8 JANUARY, THURSDAY

Avoid fruits and nuts. You are what you eat.
— Jim Davis

Aloe, banana, walnuts, probiotics, supplements, herbs, tofu, Numi honeybush tea, 3 halves artichoke hearts (canned in water), Persian dal (w/tofu, Beluga black lentil sprouts in a bed of shredded raw cabbage), aloe, green juice, Nascent Iodine.

Got up and dressed today. Had a cup of coffee w/soy milk. 70% energy level.

From: esp <espbooks@gmail.com>
Date: Thu, Jan 8, 2015 at 8:55 AM
Subject: Re: Antibiotic-induced colitis, *C. diff* infection
To: Sharon

Hello Sharon
Another question. A friend brought over some VSL#3 probiotics to help out with my *C. difficile* and colitis.

https://www.drmcdougall.com/misc/2005nl/august/050800pro.htm
I found this list on the webpage:
Ulcerative Colitis:
Escherichia coli, Nissle strain (1917)
BIFICO (3 *Bifidobacteria* species)
Saccharomyces boulardii
VLS 3 brand (*Lactobacillus and Bifidobacteria*)

Dr. McDougall's recommendations.

The VSL#3 is a milk-based product.

I found this on the VSL#3 website:

VSL#3 products may contain trace amounts of lactose [0.1g per 100g] and dehydrated skim milk or milk protein (casein and beta-lacto globulin of less than 2mg/Kg).

Any feedback on this? It's a dairy product.

thank you for your time and attention

enJOY
ellen
END EMAIL

Claudio goes to Big Sur for a work-related activity. I go along for the ride. First road trip, other than doctor stuff. I do good. I get tired but it is good to be out.

EMAIL
From: Sharon
Date: Thu, Jan 8, 2015 at 3:04 PM
Subject: RE: Antibiotic-induced colitis, *C. diff* infection
To: esp <espbooks@gmail.com>

Look for a probiotic without dairy products. There are many available. Go to your local Whole Foods (or other natural food store) and ask for their help in finding one.
Sharon
END EMAIL

EMAIL
From: <espbooks@gmail.com>
Date: Thu, Jan 8, 2015 at 3:17 PM
Subject: Re: Antibiotic-induced colitis, *C. diff* infection
To: Sharon

Thank you Sharon

That was my sense.
But Dr McDougall recommended it in the old newsletter i found and gave reference to the VSL#3. Just checking.

I am trying to gain weight now, finding it a challenge.

enJOY
ellen
END EMAIL

9 JANUARY, FRIDAY *100.3 pounds*

Chronic disease is a foodborne illness. We ate our way into this mess, and we must eat our way out.

— Mark Hyman

Aloe, probiotics, Bio-K+ (50 billion rice fermented dairy-free probiotic), supplements, herbs, amaranth, walnuts, banana, cinnamon, agave, coffee w/coconut milk, apple, Trader Joe's Force Primeval Bars (raisin/walnut/apple bars), falafel salad w/tahini dressing.

Bio-K+ 50 billion rice fermented dairy-free probiotic
https://www.biokplus.com/en_ca/products/organic-rice

93% energy level. - Day Two trying to get normal.
I found the company for the Italian licorice (an anti-bacterial): http://thelicoricecompany.com
Licorice:
http://www.acs.org/content/acs/en/pressroom/presspacs/2012/acs-presspac-february-22-2012/dried-licorice-root-fights-the-bacteria-that-cause-tooth-decay-and-gum-disease.html

https://www.drmcdougall.com/health/education/videos/mcdougalls-moments **McDougall's Moments: Short video lessons from Dr. McDougall**
****
Went to a movie, *Night at the Museum 3*. Silly but I laughed. Nice to go out and not have to panic and find the toilet. I eat a bit of Kettle corn but sense that the sharp kernel shells might irritate or scrape my colon lining. BIG night out. Trader Joe's Force Primeval Bars raisin/walnut/apple bars.

10 JANUARY, SATURDAY *101.4 pounds*

Aloe, supplements, herbs, herb tea, banana, 2 brown rice cakes/tahini, leftover Persian dal w/lentil sprouts, Blueberry Cherry Kevita, Quinoa pasta (w/olives artichoke hearts, raw garlic), gluten-free ginger cookies.

96/57 blood pressure 71 heart beat.

http://www.ncbi.nlm.nih.gov/pubmed/77366
Clostridium difficile and the aetiology of pseudomembranous colitis.

http://www.ncbi.nlm.nih.gov/pmc/articles/PMC2679968/
Toxin B is essential for virulence of *Clostridium difficile*

EMAIL
From: esp <espbooks@gmail.com>
Date: Sat, Jan 10, 2015 at 10:45 AM
Subject: Re: Antibiotic-induced colitis, *C. diff* infection
To: Sharon

Hello Sharon

again, thank you so much.

I am not gaining weight but lost two pounds eating one avocado/day and some walnuts. Three days ago I started eating tofu and soy milk, hoping to chub up. Shall I start coconut milk? Dr. McDougall doesn't recommend it, right? . . . because of the fat. I got out of bed yesterday and wore myself out.
thank you
ellen
END EMAIL

From: esp <espbooks@gmail.com>
Date: Sat, Jan 10, 2015 at 5:57 PM
Subject: antibacterial plants
To: Sharon

Hi Sharon

How do antibacterial plants (such as garlic, oregano, cinnamon) not kill the good gut bacteria. Or do they?

thank you,
ellen

11 JANUARY, MONDAY *102 pounds*

Lynne calls with an enzyme dream involving me that she had last night.

Bio-K+ 50 billion rice fermented probiotics, banana, apple, Trader Joe's Force Primeval Bars, walnuts, cashews, olive tapenade raw pizza, enzymes, ...

12 JANUARY, MONDAY *103 pounds*

BioK+ rice fermented probiotic, banana . . . . Trader Joe's Force Primeval Bars, Rooibus tea w/soy milk, rice cracker w/tahini, Wellness herb tea, Potato & Corn Chowder w/coconut milk, green juice w/fiber.

Good bowel movement!!!! Almost there!!!!

EMAIL
From: Sharon
Date: Mon, Jan 12, 2015 at 9:13 AM
Subject: RE: Antibiotic-induced colitis, *C. diff* infection
To: esp <espbooks@gmail.com>

No coconut milk yet. Too much saturated fat.

END EMAIL

13 JANUARY, TUESDAY *103.4 pounds*

Bio-K+ 50 billion rice fermented probiotic, supplements, colloidal silver, herbs, enzymes, Blueberry Cherry Kevita, cashews, 2 Trader Joe's Force Primeval Bars, apple, 2 rice crackers w/tahini, black tea chai w/almond milk, Potato Corn Chowder w/shredded raw cabbage, basil, and no-parmesan cheese (nutritional yeast/almond flour).

LETTER (handwritten):
Hello DDS

I am still in bed recovering from the antibiotic-induced colitis. I intend to get retested for the C. difficile toxins. From what I am reading, relapses are not uncommon. This terrifies me as I felt that I could have died. My life has changed and, except for a bad tooth, I was a very healthy human. I am a backpacker and spent last August

73

in the Sierra backpacking solo.

I have been studying bacteriophage therapy. Four strains of *C. difficile* have been found. Currently a phage has not been found for *C. difficile*. Hopefully a phage will be discovered. This is promising but many years in the future.

I have been taking probiotics and sent some to my children and grandchildren since I cooked Christmas dinner for everyone. At that time I did not know about the clindamycin/colitis/*C. difficile* connection and that I might be giving them the gift of diarrhea/colitis/*C. difficile*. This has been emotionally and physically traumatic and exhausting. I have enclosed photocopies of lab tests, info and notes.

I would like a refund of $1622.00 put back on my credit card. I am not a satisfied customer. I appreciate that you told me about the black tea. Thank you. Otherwise I am not happy or healthy.

Ellen Pendleton
END LETTER

16 JANUARY, FRIDAY

http://www.health-science-spirit.com/candida.html ~Candida

Herxheimer reaction

Lugol's iodine treatment with MMS

http://www.health-science-spirit.com/iodine.html
IODINE ~ Bring Back the Universal Nutrient Medicine
http://www.naturalnews.com/022800.html ~ **Iodine**

20 JANUARY, TUESDAY *103.4 pounds*

Enzymes, probiotics, banana

21 JANUARY, WEDNESDAY *103.4 pounds*

To heal from the inside out is the key.
— Wynonna Judd

I dress, go outside and water the buckthorn trees up by the road and spend 1-½ hours outside. Sweet. Sunshine recommends drinking a gallon of water every day, so I get out a glass half gallon jug to dedicate for water use.

My spirit comes in for a landing.
****
https://www.youtube.com/watch?v=mOmELsbGYYY
Video ~   Dr. Reveals Amazing Fluoride Cleanse

http://www.globalhealingcenter.com/ab/cre/detoxadine/dt_v1.html?utm_content=2320053452&utm_term=nascent%20iodine&utm_campaign=Detoxadine&utm_source=Bing_Yahoo&utm_medium=cpc
Detoxadine® - Nascent Iodine Supplement
****

Dr. Group Nascent Iodine ~ I take this daily now.

22 January, Thursday *104 pounds*

23 January, Friday *104.6 pounds, chubbing up*

Banana, coffee, Trader Joe's Force Primeval Bars, ...
I read the ingredients for these apple/raisin/walnut bars
and it doesn't say "whole wheat flour" but rather "wheat
flour," which doesn't mean, "whole wheat flour." Darn.
It's white wheat flour. Done.

24 January, Saturday

I am not getting healthy, feeling weak, going to bed early,
laying around all day. I took a little Soberanes walk today,
my first in about six weeks. Big waves today and it was
beautiful weather in the 70s.
　　　While i lay here trying to go to sleep, i ask, why
am i not getting well?

Could the *C. difficile* be in my blood? I get up, put on my
glasses, turn on the computer and here I am:
http://www.ncbi.nlm.nih.gov/pmc/articles/PMC2374624/
***Clostridium difficile*: the increasingly difficult pathogen**

http://www.ncbi.nlm.nih.gov/pubmed/14599633/
***Clostridium difficile* infection in patients with unexplained
leukocytosis.**

http://en.wikipedia.org/wiki/Septic_shock **Septic shock**

http://www.ppdictionary.com/bacteria/gpbac/difficile.htm
Pathogen Profile Dictionary ~ *Clostridium difficile*

25 JANUARY, SUNDAY

http://www.c-difficile-treatment.com

This website offers a book. I have not bought it.

C. difficile treatment $27 for eBook $36 for hard copy

****
http://www.c-difficile-treatment.com/natural-solutions-for-c-diff/ **~ treatments**

http://www.c-difficile-treatment.com/reports/c-diff-report-10-things-rev-2-1.pdf

26 JANUARY, TUESDAY

It is time to get well. Claudio is on the phone in his office and i hear him talking about me and my backpacking adventures: "... and she's just a little thing but badass!"

The only badass thing about me right now is my colon. I want to be able to do what I did last August again. That was a badass trip. And I was awesome and had an incredible time. It is time to get well so I can GO OUT AND PLAY, damn it.

What do I need to get well? What?

Phage Workers. In 1960 James Watson received the Eli Lilly Award in Biological Chemistry then it appears that he stopped researching phages.

http://en.wikipedia.org/wiki/Eli_Lilly_Award_in_Biological_C hemistry

his website:

http://www.cshl.edu/gradschool/james-d-watson.html

CSHLPress: http://www.cshlpress.com/ ~ cshpress@cshl.edu

http://jama.jamanetwork.com/article.aspx?articleid=1484499

Found it:
Eradicating *C difficile*

Tracy Hampton, PhD

JAMA. 2012;308(22):2326. doi:10.1001/jama.2012.111751.
http://jama.jamanetwork.com/article.aspx?
articleid=1484499#tab1
A combination of 6 naturally occurring bacteria can eradicate a highly contagious form of *Clostridium difficile* in mice (Lawley TD et al. *PLoS Pathog.* 2012;8[10]:e1002995). The mix included 3 previously described species (*Staphylococcus warneri*, *Enterococcus hirae*, and *Lactobacillus reuteri*) and 3 novel species.

Mice in the study were infected with a persistent form of *C difficile* that consistently relapsed to a high level of shedding or contagiousness after the animals were treated with a range of antibiotics.

Staphylococcus warneri

http://www.ncbi.nlm.nih.gov/pubmed/13677632

Enterococcus hirae

http://www.ncbi.nlm.nih.gov/pmc/articles/PMC3524446/

Lactobacillus reuteri

http://en.wikipedia.org/wiki/Lactobacillus_reuteri
**H

m-m-m. This is ringing my Truth-O-Meter. Is *L. reuteri* available?

****
http://phickle.com/index.php/rejuvelac-the-healthiest-ferment/ ~ **Fermented Sprout Drink Rejuvelac**

Sprout Chart: http://www.vegetariantimes.com/blog/how-to-soak-and-sprout-nuts-seeds-grains-and-beans

http://phickle.com/index.php/rejuvelac-the-healthiest-ferment/

Carrot Spice Kombucha
http://phickle.com/index.php/category/vegan/

Kombucha tea ~ www.getkombucha.com/kombucha-benefits/

After dinner Claudio and I drive to CVS and Whole Foods to find the *Lactobacillus reuteri* and do. Nature's Way®, Primodophilus® Reuteri, 5 billion CFU/90 Vcaps®. CFU = Colony Forming Unit.

27 JANUARY, TUESDAY **105 pounds**

28 JANUARY, WEDNESDAY **106 pounds**

https://www.youtube.com/watch?v=5Zi2Rl-bI7E

EndoLISA® Endotoxin Detection - English language
~ this is a curious video on lab testing.

29 JANUARY THURSDAY *105.2 pounds*

http://phage-biotech.com/ ~ **Israel**

Contact

G. Eliava Institute of Bacteriophages, Microbiology and Virology
3, Gotua str., Tbilisi 0160, Georgia
Tel: +995 322 37 4910
Director: Dr. Mzia Kutateladze
Tel: +995 322 381604 Fax: +995 322 374910
E-mail: kutateladze@pha.ge

Deputy Director: David Asatiani
Tel/fax: +995 322 379410
d110ani@gmail.com

EMAIL
E-mail: d110ani@gmail.com
Greetings

Have you found a phage for *C. difficile*?

My lab test detected Toxigenic *C. difficile* on Dec. 27 and I would like to try phage therapy. But apparently, the phage has not been found.

any clues?

thank you

Ellen Pendleton

END EMAIL

http://www.ncbi.nlm.nih.gov/pmc/articles/PMC90351/

2014 white paper ~ Bacteriophage Therapy

http://ehp.niehs.nih.gov/121-a48/ **Phage Renaissance: New Hope against Antibiotic Resistance**

http://informahealthcare.com/doi/abs/10.3109/08910609509 141381 ~ **Safety and Tolerance of *Lactobacillus reuteri* in Healthy Adult Male Subjects. Read More:** http://informahealthcare.com/doi/abs/10.3109/08910609509 141381

Production of a Broad Spectrum Antimicrobial Substance by *Lactobacillus reuteri* Read More: http://informahealthcare.com/doi/abs/10.3109/08910608909 140210?src=recsys

30 JANUARY, FRIDAY *103 pounds*

1 FEBRUARY, SUPERBOWL SUNDAY *102.6 POUNDS*

Lynne and Michael join us for SuperBowl and bring a lovely green salad with a no-oil dressing. I solar bake a black lentil dal tagine. Michael introduces me to apples dipped in tahini. Yippee!

After the game and after they leave, my gut has some cramps and wrenches. My sense is that it might have been the black caraway seeds that I sprinkled on top of the cooked tagine. They didn't get a chance to soften and could have been hard on my colon lining.

3 February, Tuesday

http://jmm.sgmjournals.org/content/54/2/129.abstract
Slovenia phage therapy

http://mic.sgmjournals.org/content/153/3/676.abstract

The complete genome sequence of *Clostridium difficile* phage φC2 and comparisons to φCD119 and inducible prophages of CD630

4 February, Wednesday *103.6 pounds*

The soul is healed by being with children.
> — Fyodor Dostoyevsky

Abdominal cramps. No energy. I do not want a relapse.
http://www.jafral.com/en/ ~ **phage therapy in Slovenia**

https://www5.vetmed.auburn.edu/~petreva/Files/EPC_Program.pdf ~ **Edinburgh International Phage Conference 2008**
****

My youngest granddaughter is having her birthday celebration at the bowling alley. I go, expecting a huge input of energy and there is. I conserve my energy, keep a smile on my face and survive. I would LOVE to bowl a few games but I do not wish to push it. I'd probably have to pay tomorrow.

5 February, Thursday *103 pounds*

L. reuteri, aloe. Going back to mono eating. Probiotics

individually too; some may work against each other and the antibacterial foods and herbs. Brown rice w/Dr. Braggs Liquid Aminos, tea w/almond milk, banana, almond meal, walnuts, tea, brown rice/lentil casserole w/spinach & carrots, Bio-K+ fermented rice probiotic, Kevita, bowl of TJ Toasted Oatmeal cereal w/soy milk.

http://www.healingwell.com/community/default.aspx?f=38&m=1241671 Clindamycin HCl **HealingWell.com Forum**

https://www.millerandzois.com/four-mistakes-that-lead-to-c-difficle-lawsuits.html
Four Mistakes that lead to *C. Difficle* Lawsuits

****

http://www.rxlist.com/imodium-drug/overdosage-contraindications.htm ~ **Imodium contraindications**

— in patients with pseudomembranous colitis associated with the use of broad-spectrum antibiotics.

http://www.naturalhealthadvisory.com/daily/natural-health-101/c-diff-symptoms-and-treatments/
***C-Diff* Symptoms and Treatments**

6 FEBRUARY, FRIDAY

Bio-K+ fermented rice probiotic, ...

8 FEBRUARY, SUNDAY
MEDICINAL INDIAN HUMMUS

"Okay," you say. "Is that why you're not healthy?" responding to my whole food, plant-based diet choice.

No. That's why I am getting well. I am not well yet, still in my bathrobe, still doing what I know to do to get well and trying my best to be patient. *Doctors Practice; We are Patient.*

LETTER
To: Alpha Books
800 East 96th Street
Indianapolis, IN 46240

Hello Alpha Books

I am writing a book regarding my personal healing process from antibiotic-induced pseudomembranous colitis and *Clostridium difficile*. One of my favorite healing foods is based on the Indian Hummus recipe, page 273 in your book, *The Complete Idiot's Guide to Plant-Based Nutrition* by Julieanna Hever. I make a few modifications adding more turmeric, garlic, etc.

I would like your permission to put the recipe in my book. Do I need it? How do I go about obtaining it?

Thank you and enJOY life,
Ellen Pendleton
END LETTER

9 FEBRUARY, MONDAY *103.4 pounds*
BLACK TEA

Your failure to be informed does not make me a wacko.
— John Loeffler

Bio-K+ fermented rice probiotic, ...

I am sitting here looking at the bottle of clindamycin on my desk, nine capsules left. If a lab test could be done on these capsules, would the *Clostridium difficile* bacteria be present in the capsules??? Nothing would surprise me now. The instructions always say to complete the dosage. This destroys the evidence. Food for fiction.

****

http://www.drugs.com/manufacturer/ranbaxy-pharmaceuticals-inc-120.html
Ranbaxy Pharmaceuticals Inc.

http://www.drugs.com/pro/clindamycin-capsules.html
To reduce the development of drug-resistant bacteria and maintain the effectiveness of clindamycin HCl and other antibacterial drugs, clindamycin HCl should be used only to treat or prevent infections that are proven or strongly suspected to be caused by bacteria.
www.drugs.com/sfx/clindamycin-side-effects.html
For Healthcare Professionals
Applies to clindamycin: compounding powder, injectable solution, intravenous solution, oral capsule, oral powder for reconstitution

Gastrointestinal

The onset of pseudomembranous colitis symptoms may occur during or after antibacterial treatment and is associated with the presence of *Clostridium difficile* toxin in the stool. Pseudomembranous colitis may also be associated with toxic megacolon, which can be life-threatening.

References http://www.ncbi.nlm.nih.gov/pubmed/12523467
1. de Groot MC, van Puijenbroek EP **"Clindamycin and taste disorders."** Br J Clin Pharmacol 64 (2007): 542-5
2. Meadowcroft AM, Diaz PR, Latham GS **"Clostridium difficile**

toxin-induced colitis after use of clindmycin phosphate vaginal cream." Ann Pharmacother 32 (1998): 309-11

3. Davies J, Beck E **"Recurrent colitis following antibiotic-associated pseudomembranous colitis."** Postgrad Med J 57 (1981): 599-601

4. Milstone EB, McDonald AJ, Scholhamer CF Jr **"Pseudomembranous colitis after topical application of clindamycin."** Arch Dermatol 117 (1981): 154-5

5. Bartlett JG **"Narrative review: the new epidemic of *Clostridium difficile*-associated enteric disease."** Ann Intern Med 145 (2006): 758-64

6. Cerner Multum, Inc. **"Australian Product Information."** O 0

7. Leigh DA, Simmons K, Williams S **"Gastrointestinal side effects following clindamycin and lincomycin treatment: a follow up study."** J Antimicrob Chemother 6 (1980): 639-45

8. George WL, Sutter VL, Finegold SM **"Antimicrobial agent-induced diarrhea--a bacterial disease."** J Infect Dis 136 (1977): 822-8

9. Cerner Multum, Inc. **UK Summary of Product Characteristics.** O 0

10. Wilson DH **"Clindamycin in the treatment of soft tissue infections: a review of 15,019 patients."** Br J Surg 67 (1980): 93-6

11. Mason SJ, O'Meara TF **"Drug-induced esophagitis."** J Clin Gastroenterol 3 (1981): 115-20

12. Geddes AM, Bridgwater FA, Williams DN, Oon J, Grimshaw GJ **"Clinical and bacteriological studies with clindamycin."** Br Med J 2 (1970): 703-4

13. Parry MF, Rha CK **"Pseudomembranous colitis caused by topical clindamycin phosphate."** Arch Dermatol 122 (1986): 583-4

14. Van Ness MM, Cattau EL Jr **"Fulminant colitis complicating antibiotic-associated pseudomembranous colitis: case report and review of the clinical manifestations and treatment."** Am J Gastroenterol 82 (1987): 374-7

15. Cone JB, Wetzel W **"Toxic megacolon secondary to pseudomembranous colitis."** Dis Colon Rectum 25 (1982): 478-82

16. **"Product Information. Cleocin (clindamycin)."** Pharmacia and Upjohn, Kalamazoo, MI.

17. Clark BM, Homeyer DC, Glass KR, D'Avignon LC **"Clindamycin-Induced Sweet's Syndrome."** Pharmacotherapy 27

(2007): 1343-6

18. Vidal C, Iglesias A, Saez A, Rodriguez M **"Hypersensitivity to clindamycin."** DICP 25 (1991): 317

19. Kapoor R, Flynn C, Heald PW, Kapoor JR **"Acute generalized exanthematous pustulosis induced by clindamycin."** Arch Dermatol 142 (2006): 1080-1

20. Miller Quidley A, Bookstaver PB, Gainey AB, Gainey MD **"Fatal clindamycin-induced drug rash with eosinophilia and systemic symptoms (DRESS) syndrome."** Pharmacotherapy (2012):

21. Tian D, Mohan RJ, Stallings G **"Drug rash with eosinophilia and systemic symptoms syndrome associated with clindamycin."** Am J Med 123 (2010): e7-8

22. Paquet P, Schaaflafontaine N, Pierard GE **"Toxic epidermal necrolysis following clindamycin treatment."** Br J Dermatol 132 (1995): 665-6

23. Lammintausta K, Tokola R, Kalimo K **"Cutaneous adverse reactions to clindamycin: results of skin tests and oral exposure."** Br J Dermatol 146 (2002): 643-8

24. Bubalo JS, Blasdel CS, Bearden DT **"Neutropenia after single-dose clindamycin for dental prophylaxis."** Pharmacotherapy 23 (2003): 101-3

****

I intend to follow-up on all of these reference footnotes listed but right now I have to find a mouse in the house. It ran across the hallway into my office and I closed the door behind it. Then I put in some poison. I was not in the mood to catch it and I don't have a *"**Have A Heart**"* trap.

That was a week ago so now I am taking apart my office, . . . everything, looking for a mouse, dead or alive. I find a hole low in the closet wall where it might have escaped into who-knows-where. I tape it up with duct tape.

In the search and cleaning of my office, I find a CD that was given as a Christmas gift from Annie and Paul that, in all of this intestinal mayhem, I forgot about. I really haven't been up and around much since the shit hit the fan. Annie and Paul made the CD and is in a hand-written envelope. I put on the CD and it opens with an audio greeting by Annie, then Indian flute music divine. I get the phone and immediately call Annie to tell her the whole story of what has happened since Christmas. And here's why I write about this: I tell her about the black tea stopping the diarrhea.

"Black tea has a lot of fluoride in it," she says. And Annie is some kind of doctor, maybe a psychiatrist?

"Really? I did not know that."

We talk a good talk and as it turns out she's got some colon/rectum issues going on. She called it Irritable Bowel Syndrome and she's got a fissure, a gaping tear. Lots to share.

I am now looking up keywords: **black tea fluoride:**
http://www.sciencedaily.com/releases/2010/07/100714104059.htm
Tea may contain more fluoride than once thought, research shows ~ Science Daily
Most published reports show 1 to 5 milligrams of fluoride per liter of black tea, but a new study shows that number could be as high as 9 milligrams.
Fluoride is known to help prevent dental cavities, but long-term ingestion of excessive amounts could cause bone problems.
***[

AUTHOR'S NOTE — *Fluoride is known to help prevent dental cavities,* is a CONTROVERSIAL STATEMENT]

****

Evidently the tea plant sucks up aluminum and fluoride from the soil into the leaves. Guess that does it for black tea.

****

Can probiotics reduce severity of *C. difficile* infections?
www.sciencedaily.com/releases/2014/08/140807215529.htm

C. difficile colonization accompanied by changes in gut microbiota: Study hints at probiotics as treatment
http://www.sciencedaily.com/releases/2011/04/110419214849.htm

This is an excellent video: https://vimeo.com/99575315
Emma Allen-Vercoe, PhD (2014) The gut microbiota and why it is important in ASD.
It's a half an hour in length but worth the time.

Vercoe refers to working with Martin Blaser, http://martinblaser.com and here's his quick video off of his website: https://www.youtube.com/watch?v=3ew37rxAhjg
Dr. Martin Blaser Introduces 'Missing Microbes'

This is a favorite: The gut flora: You and your 100 trillion friends: Jeroen Raes at TEDxBrussels
https://www.youtube.com/watch?v=Af5qUxl1ktI
Jeroen Raes says it could take a year to reflourish the gut flora, or maybe never. OMG. NEVER? Great video.

This is interesting:
http://www.sciencedaily.com/releases/2011/04/110419214849.htm
C. difficile colonization accompanied by changes in gut microbiota: Study hints at probiotics as treatment

Clostridium difficile Colonization in Early Infancy Is Accompanied by Changes in Intestinal Microbiota Composition

****

Some herbals and supplements for intestinal care:
http://www.renewlife.com/specialty-supplements/intestinew.html

10 FEBRUARY, TUESDAY *103.8 pounds*
ENERGY SHIFT

Life is a combination of magic and pasta.
                    — Federico Fellini

Coffee, aspirin, ...

I wake up, lay in bed and meditate for a long time, get up, go pee, weigh myself, 103.8 pounds, drink some aloe, take some probiotics and go back to bed. That's it. That's all I've got. After his breakfast Claudio comes in and asks, "Okay. What is your energy level?"

"Forty percent."

"This is the lowest you've been. You worked too hard yesterday," and he scolds me. I know that he's afraid and concerned but I don't have much energy to respond. This is not my best day.

I drink coffee instead of tea, knowing that it is probably not the best for my gut but I miss coffee and the caffeine pick-me-up. It takes two cups and still, it doesn't do the magic. I put some potatoes out to solar bake and study more.

****

http://www.ihaveuc.com/author/timo-cavalheiro-liesimaa/
Timo Cavalheiro Liesimaa

http://www.ihaveuc.com/four-positive-changes-for-managing-uc/ **Four Positive Changes for Managing UC**

EMAILS
Scout: Say can you go for walks yet? How about a shorty at Pt. Lobos on Wednesday. Coming in to work at Flanders.

mi: Yes, come on by. I'll see about a walk. Haven't yet. Yesterday i wore myself out looking for a mouse in my office. Haven't found it yet. Have to put the office back together today and find places for all the other stuff i don't want to put back in.

Scout: I'll come by Wednesday. Rest up. We can try a short walk if you're up for it.
END EMAILS

I can't imagine taking a walk.

Late afternoon my shoulder, neck and head hurt so I take two aspirin. I find this:
https://www.herbdoc.com/blog/book/there-are-no-incurable-diseases ~ I ordered but haven't received the Dr. Schulze *Incurables* book yet so I get back onto the website and look it up. It is available eBook.

Time to read. It won't let me download it so I have to read it on the computer (not my favorite).

My energy level is much higher and I suggest we go out to dinner. We do and I'm feeling renewed.

mi: okay, the day started pretty crappy (excuse the pun).
but since black tea has fluoride and aluminum in it, i had a cup of coffee.
Still the day was zero energy and crappy.
Late this afternoon my shoulder, neck and head hurt so I took two aspirin.
As I did more Internet research, I came across a quote that plugged me in spiritually to heal. Be it the coffee, the aspirin, the power plug, or the thought of going for a walk with you tomorrow, I am feeling the best that I have felt since November!!! It is my spiritual duty to get well.

What time tomorrow?
i am eager to see you, Scout!

Scout: Hey energizer bunny. Is 11 ok?

mi: Perfect!
I hope I can keep this rollin'
END EMAIL

Scout is my backpacking buddy. She's good! She's great! We've been on a couple of good backpacks together. We plan to walk the *Camino de Santiago* in Spain next year.

I read more of the *There is No Incurable Disease* and feel like I have been reunited with my healing self. Thank you, Richard Schulze. Your enthusiasm is contagious. My spirit has moved into gear. With God, everything is.

****

http://blogs.naturalnews.com/4-probiotic-foods-bulletproof-immune-system/

4 Probiotic Foods that Bulletproof the Immune System
By Mayimina
Posted Thursday, December 18, 2014 at 11:44am EST

Fermented vegetables (kimchi), kefir, kombucha, apple cider vinegar.

****

I drink a glass of water with about 1/4 cup of apple cider vinegar before going to bed.

11 FEBRUARY, WEDNESDAY *102.6 pounds*

What you need is a good, two-hour walk.
　　　　　　– Jim Casteel

Coffee, aspirin. To walk or not to walk? Scout is on her way over and I haven't gotten out of my bathrobe yet. It is 11:05 a.m. Lemme check my emails.

　　I am still in my bathrobe when Scout arrives, still not sure how I'll feel. We sit in the living room and chat but the beautiful sunny day calls, so we move to the patio and enJOY the vitamin D. After about an hour I change into walking clothes and off we go down the hill for a neighborhood walk rather than Point Lobos. The walk is lovely with a few dizzy spells, weird stomach and slow moving. But it is good to be with Scout and with Mother Nature. We talk of many things and of our *Camino de Santiago* adventure. Deborah, a neighbor from up the road, drives by and I invite her to come walk the *Camino* with us next year.

In an attempt to get permission, this author catches my attention: http://blogs.naturalnews.com/author/sofiya/

Lots of good information here. I'm gonna go drink some more apple cider vinegar.

http://blogs.naturalnews.com/the-reality-of-fluoroquinolones-or-how-i-became-disabled-over-night/
The Reality of Fluoroquinolones- or- How I Became Disabled overnight

I was just looking for a white bean hummus recipe in my *Prevent and Reverse Heart Disease* book by Dr. Caldwell Esselstyn and found the insert from Metronidazole 500 Mg Tab Acta (Flagyl) that I got when I picked it up from the pharmacy. It gives the GENERIC NAME, COMMON USES, then it reads, BEFORE USING THIS MEDICINE: WARNING: Long-term use of this medicine has caused cancer in mice and rats.

Well, there it is.

Found this blog while editing:
http://sci.rutgers.edu/forum/showthread.php?6313-Clostridium-difficile-diarrhea ~ These blogs are scary, "My mom went into the hospital for ankle surgery, got diarrhea from an intestinal bacteria, CDIFF, and died."

12 FEBRUARY, THURSDAY **104.2 pounds**

You are what you eat. For example, if you eat garlic you're apt to be a hermit. — Franklin P. Jones

Black tea w/almond milk, banana, avocado, rice cakes w/Kalamata olive, white bean, raw garlic, hummus.

Had a busy morning with the downstairs studio apartment and pushed some furniture around. Now I am tired.

Claudio receives some emails from a business associate in Texas and comes in to read the latest one out loud.

EMAILS
> From: rick
> Date: Thu, 12 Feb 2015 00:22:37 -0600
> Subject: Call
> To: CW
>
> C.W.,
>
> Sorry I missed your call, the message you left didn't come thru but I'm sure you're wanting a update. Thank God I am still alive despite the multiple complications I had with my hip replacement. Last year was truly a trial as I spent 3 weeks in the hospital at various times due to the intestinal bacteria I got that was antibiotic resistant. Over 20,000 people in the US died last year from this same bacteria. I can now say the bacteria is dead and I am the winner after 12 months of hell.
>
> I have completed the construction on a couple of projects and have them on the market for sale. Once I close one of these I will be able to send you funds again. Sorry for the delay but with all I've been through I have literally done the best I could to keep things going and recover from this nightmare. I hope all is well with you and that 2015 brings us all a time of refreshing and prosperity.
> Best regards,
> Rick

On Feb 12, 2015, at 1:00 AM, C.W. wrote:

Hi Rick

Thanks for the update. I'm glad you are recovering. My partner took an antibiotic prescribed by her dentist and she got colitis with the bacteria c dificil[sp]. This has put her in bed for the last 2 months. She won't take any more antibiotics, so she is self treating by a strict vegan diet with tons of probiotics.

Is this the bacteria you got? Did you have to take other antibiotics to get rid of it? This thing is evil. You are lucky to have beaten it.

Be well,
CW

From: rick
Subject: Re: Call
Date: Thu, 12 Feb 2015 12:06:45 -0600

C.W.

It is C-Diff that I got and the insurance required me to do the traditional treatments of antibiotics, but every time I finished a course of the antibiotic within a few days the C-Diff took over again. Finally after 10 months of Hell the FDA approved a new antibiotic to specifically treat this bacteria. It cost $4,000.00 for ten days but it finally killed the bug and I have been slowly regaining my strength. There is a probiotic called Florastor that helps relieve the toxic gas that is put off by the C-Diff bacteria.

I hope she gets well soon, I know how terrible this bacteria can be.

Best regards,
Rick
END EMAIL

Interesting. Florastor, lemme look it up.

Product Description - Amazon.com

Florastor *saccharomyces boulardii lyo*, florastor contain the active ingredient *saccharomyces boulardii lyo*, a non-pathogenic yeast found naturally on the skin of tropical fruit (lychee and

96

mangosteens). Florastor helps support healthy digestive system. Florastor also acts to maintain the balance of intestinal flora.

[NOTE: mangosteen again]

Florastor manufactured by Biocodex.
http://www.biocodexusa.com/
Our flagship product, **Florastor®** (*Saccharomyces boulardii lyo*), is available at major retail pharmacies throughout the United States.

I am already taking Saccharomyces boulardii.

Fidaxomicin ~ http://www.dificid.com/
Lemme look up the side effects (besides the cost).
Please see full Prescribing Information for DIFICID.

http://www.dificid.com/downloads/Dificid_PI.pdf

ADVERSE REACTIONS

The most common adverse reactions are nausea (11%), vomiting (7%), abdominal pain (6%), gastrointestinal hemorrhage (4%), anemia (2%), and neutropenia (2%).

I am not feeling lucky. 4% gastrointestial hemorrhage, 2% neutropenia. I am not sure what neutropenia but it sounds devastating.

http://en.wikipedia.org/wiki/Neutropenia

Neutropenia or **neutropaenia**, from Latin prefix *neutro-* ("neither", for neutral staining) and Greek suffix -πενία (*-penía*, "deficiency"), is a granulocyte disorder characterized by an abnormally low number of neutrophils. Neutrophils usually make up 60 to 70% of circulating white blood cells and serve as the primary defense against infections by destroying bacteria in the blood. Hence, patients with neutropenia are more susceptible to bacterial infections and, without prompt medical attention, the condition may become

97

life-threatening and deadly (neutropenic sepsis).

6.2 Post Marketing Experience
Adverse reactions reported in the post marketing setting arise from a population of unknown size and are voluntary in nature. As such,
reliability in estimating their frequency or in establishing a causal relationship to drug exposure is not always possible.
Hypersensitivity reactions (dyspnea, angioedema, rash, and pruritus) have been reported

Dyspnea

http://www.medicinenet.com/script/main/art.asp?
articlekey=3145 **Dyspnea:** Difficult or labored breathing; shortness of breath. Dyspnea is a sign of serious disease of the airway, lungs, or heart. The onset of dyspnea should not be ignored; it is reason to seek medical attention.

Angioedema ~ http://en.wikipedia.org/wiki/Angioedema

Angioedema (BE: **angiooedema**) or **Quincke's edema** is the rapid swelling (edema) of the dermis, subcutaneous tissue,[1] mucosa and submucosal tissues. It is very similar to urticaria, but urticaria, commonly known as hives, occurs in the upper dermis.[1] The term **angioneurotic oedema** was used for this condition in the belief that there was nervous system involvement, but this is no longer thought to be the case.

Pruritus
http://emedicine.medscape.com/article/1098029-overview
Pruritus and Systemic Disease ~ Pruritus, or itch, is defined as an unpleasant sensation that provokes the desire to scratch. Certain systemic diseases have long been known to cause pruritus that ranges in intensity from a mild annoyance to an intractable, disabling condition. Generalized pruritus may be classified into the following categories on the basis of the underlying causative disease: renal pruritus, cholestatic pruritus, hematologic pruritus, endocrine pruritus, pruritus related to malignancy, and idiopathic generalized pruritus.

Yesterday I made a vegan Lavender Cheesecake to give Edie for her birthday today. I had to cancel my appointment with her due to the downstairs studio incident that required my attention. She won't be back in town till Wednesday and I planned to save the cheesecake for her. But tonight, for dessert, Claudio, Tom and I each have a piece and it is good.

Now it's bedtime and my gut is gurgling. Coconut oil. I didn't make the cheesecake for me and didn't intend to eat any of it but couldn't resist. I haven't had oil like this in my gut since way before I got sick. Gurgling. Too much oil. What shall I take? Rice milk? I'll probably weigh more in the morning.

http://www.phagetherapycenter.com
I do a Mapquest search on the **Eliava Institute in Tbilisi, Georgia** and it looks fascinating.

EMAIL:
mailbox@phagetherapycenter.com
Greetings

I am willing to travel to Georgia for phage therapy treatment. Do you have a phage yet for *Clostridium difficile?*

Toxigenic *C. difficile* was detected on my lab test dated 27 Dec 2014. The diarrhea has stopped. I am trying to recover but would like to have phage therapy treatment.

I am writing a book about my path to recovery and looking for a happy ending.

Thank you
Ellen Pendleton
END EMAIL

The practice of forgiveness is our most important contribution to the healing of the world. — Marianne Williamson

EMAIL:
Dear Ellen,

Unfortunately there are currently no therapeutic phages for treating *C. difficile*.

There is a protocol that sometimes works, which we can offer to you. It is our experience that *C. difficile* is often accompanied by pathogenic *E.coli*. We can treat the *E.coli* and at the same time introduce a non-pathogenic strain of this bacteria that is a *C.difficile* antagonist; in other words this non-pathogenic strain of *E.coli* can kill or displace the *C.difficile*. When used in combination with probiotics and other natural medications, in many cases we can bring the flora back to normal. However, we can offer no guarantee of success.

If you are interested in this protocol, please register as our patient at www.phagetherapycenter.com and we will provide you with specific instructions.

Thank you for contacting our clinic.

With kind regards,
Giorgi Namgaladze, Patient Coordinator
Phage Therapy Center
END EMAIL

EMAIL
From: esp <espbooks@gmail.com>
Date: Fri, Feb 13, 2015 at 10:37 AM
Subject: Re: *Clostridium difficile*
To: gnamgaladze@phagetherapycenter.com

Thank you, Giorgi

Is the *E. Coli* treatment like fecal transplant?

Would I have to go to Georgia for treatment?

Best regards,
Ellen
END EMAIL

14 February, Saturday

All healing is first a healing of the heart.
— Carl Townsend

I look inside at what was going on in my life when I first noticed symptoms. My sutures were removed December 16. And also that day, Margie, my former mother-in-law, died. She was my adopted mother. My heart still hurts. There were also some issues with my children that I won't go into.

Hadn't heard of this one until now: Teicoplanin
http://www.ncbi.nlm.nih.gov/pubmed/21901692
Antibiotic treatment for *Clostridium difficile*-associated diarrhea in adults

Teicoplanin is not available in the USA. It's available in France and expensive.

15 FEBRUARY, SUNDAY

A lot of people say they want to get out of pain, and I'm sure that's true, but they aren't willing to make healing a high priority. They aren't willing to look inside to see the source of their pain in order to deal with it. – Lindsay Wagner

Food eaten: Almond meal, supplements and herbs, coffee w/soy milk.

Health Benefits of Beets:
http://foodrevolution.org/blog/health-benefits-beets/

The greatest goodness that I can do is to get well. It is my job, my responsibility, my duty, my challenge, my path to recover my well-being, continue to adventure on Planet Earth and write about it. I got it. My spirit is intact and ready to rumble. I will kick *Clostridium difficile* and live happily ever after.

Is it the coffee? Whoops.

Claudio and I drive to Santa Cruz and eat at Café Gratitude, my favorite restaurant. I order Roasted Potatoes but it has lots of oil. The restaurant is almost perfect except for the oil. I don't eat oil.

Then we wander into a sculpture gallery. My energy is still good. Claudio is amused and inspired by the works. We then find Kuumbwa Jazz Center and get into line. The concert opens with The Henhouse, all women and a male drummer. Then *The Carolyn Sills Combo* begins, with Sunshine singing harmony. The show is amazingly wonderful and I make it through the night without a gut incident!!! Sweet.

16 FEBRUARY, MONDAY **104.8 pounds**

Music is very important. It's important as a tool for learning, it can be a tool for healing, it can be no telling what, as long as we remain free to be able to create the music, to be able to experiment and to really research, and to really get time to develop the music.
— Lester Bowie

Bought some more Bio-K+ probiotics 50 billion fermented rice: *L. acidophilus* CL1285®, *L. casei* LBC80R®, and *L. rhamnosus* CLR2®. Took the last of the *L. reuteri.* Bro Tom is visiting and we watch old Tom Jones videos from the 60s or 70s on YouTube all morning. Good laughing session.

17 FEBRUARY, TUESDAY **102.8 pounds**

"Healing," Papa would tell me, "is not a science, but the intuitive art of wooing nature."
— W.H. Auden

Bio-K+, Kombucha, banana.

I get the probiotics today that I ordered:

Swanson Probiotics

http://www.swansonvitamins.com/swanson-probiotics-dr-stephen-langers-ultimate-16-strain-probioticwith-fos-60-veg-caps#label

Dr. Stephen Langer's Ultimate 16 Strain Probiotic with FOS

FOS (Fructooligosaccharides)	50 mg
ConcenTrace® Trace Mineral Complex (from the Great Salt Lake, 72 naturally occurring minerals, plus other minerals found in seawater)	12.5 mg
Bifidobacterium longum	430 million viable organisms†
Lactobacillus acidophilus	430 million viable organisms†
Bifidobacterium bifidum	180 million viable organisms†
Bifidobacterium breve	180 million viable organisms†
Bifidobacterium lactis	180 million viable organisms†
Lactobacillus brevis	180 million viable organisms†
Lactobacillus bulgaricus	180 million viable organisms†
Lactobacillus casei	180 million viable organisms†
Lactobacillus helveticus	180 million viable organisms†
Lactobacillus plantarum	180 million viable organisms†
Lactobacillus reuteri	180 million viable organisms†
Lactobacillus rhamnosus	180 million viable organisms†
Lactobacillus salivarius	180 million viable organisms†
Lactococcus lactis	180 million viable organisms†
Streptococcus thermophilus	180 million viable organisms†
Bifidobacterium infantis	90 million viable organisms†

I immediately take five capsules. Minerals are vital.

Feeling about 90% throughout the day. Gut is gurgling a bit now, almost bedtime. Maybe some peppermint and ginger tea will help.

18 FEBRUARY, WEDNESDAY

Gut issues. Down to feeling about 60% now. Not happy.
Gut cramps.

　　Wake at 3 a.m. for a Bio-K+ and water.

19 FEBRUARY, THURSDAY 104.2

*Healing is a matter of time, but it is sometimes also a matter of
opportunity.*　　　　　　— Hippocrates

No coffee this morning. Maybe the acid is irritating the
colon. I have a cup of green tea.

I put in a GoogleAlert for *difficile*. I have one alert in for
"*difficile* phage" and got about three replies. This one
comes in as soon as I sign in:
http://www.infectioncontroltoday.com/news/2015/02/scientis
ts-discover-how-c-difficile-wreaks-havoc-in-the-gut.aspx
**Scientists Discover How *C. difficile* Wreaks Havoc in the
Gut**
****
**Colonization versus carriage of *Clostridium difficile*
Infectious Disease Clinics of North America, 01/23/2015**
http://www.id.theclinics.com/article/S0891-5520(14)00078-
6/abstract?rss=yes
Asymptomatic carriage of toxigenic strains of *Clostridium difficile*
is common in health care facilities and the community.
However, infection control efforts have traditionally focused
almost entirely on symptomatic patients. There is now growing
concern that asymptomatic carriers may be an underappreciated
source of transmission. This article provides an overview of the

pathogenesis and epidemiology of *C. difficile* colonization, reviews the evidence that asymptomatic carriers shed spores and contribute to transmission, and examines practical issues related to prevention of transmission from carriers.

20 FEBRUARY, FRIDAY *104.8 pounds*

Healing yourself is connected with healing others.
— Yoko Ono

Claudio has been so concerned, supportive and helpful. I am trying! We were supposed to leave early February, traveling out of the country but the trip just didn't manifest. It turns out to be good that we didn't have flight/hotel reservations. I don't think that I would travel very well right now. I am babying my body, eating well and doing everything that I know to do to recover.

Had two cups of home-roasted organic coffee today. Let's see how this works. I am hoping the organic will be better received than the other I was drinking; too acidic.

What's next? Do I just plow through and go do things even though my energy level is at about 70%?

I haven't gotten a reply yet from the Phage Therapy Center in Georgia. Maybe I didn't send it. I'll send it again.

http://www.ncbi.nlm.nih.gov/pubmed/25626036

Diagnosis and treatment of *Clostridium difficile* in adults: a systematic review.

My sense is that I need to give Clostridium difficile a break. It might lift my spirit working on one of my fun books rather than this one. I still have much work to do on Take A Hike and The Sierra Hot Springs Walking Tour (plug, plug). It's Friday night. Maybe we'll go to a movie. Lemme C what is playing.

After the movies we pick up our mail from the post office. A priority letter is in my box from the dentist office. I open it and read the cover letter.

LETTER FROM DDS MSD:
February 16, 2015

Dear Ms. Pendleton,

I received your letter and wish to respond.
Dentistry is an art, and there are no guarantees or warranties related to a specific result. On the professional front, we have tried to deliver exceptional service and we are comfortable that our technical results would withstand any scrutiny. We are glad to confirm the success of your dental procedure in your post-operative, complimentary well checks.

You did indeed receive a prescription for clindamycin that was filled at your local pharmacy, a medication that was properly indicated for the condition we were treating. On rare occasion, a patient may develop a side effect, such as c. difficile. The warnings are always provided to you with the medications at the pharmacy, and a pharmacist is available for consultation, so you can make an educated choice of whether this medication is worth the risk. While it is not a common complication, if it happens to you, it's "100% to you." Regardless, we feel it is unfortunate you had this experience.

You have made it clear that you are less than satisfied. In order to bring this matter to a close, I am willing to tender a check for $1622. In exchange for the check you will need to sign a release form. The enclosed agreement and release form has a confidentiality provision and it is important that you read it carefully.

The payment is being offered solely as an act of good faith and good will in your health, and the exceptional care we feel we provide. You should know that refunds for dental care are virtually unheard of. If money back guarantees were the norm, our healthcare system would quickly grind to a halt. Just to be clear, the offer outlined in this letter should not be construed as any tacit or explicit admission of substandard care of customer service.

In the spirit of putting this behind us, and with my greater concern that you spend your efforts on focusing on your health, we will provide you with what you have requested. This offer will remain open for ten (10) days. There will be no other forthcoming offers. Regardless of what you decide, I wish you well.

Sincerely,
DDS MSD
END LETTER

Also included are five pages titled:

AGREEMENT

Settlement, Release, Indemnification and Hold Harmless Agreement, Ellen Pendleton

21 FEBRUARY, SATURDAY 102.8

I just read the five pages and my gut (whom I have spent the last two months nourishing and nurturing) says NO. This is a SHUT UP agreement.

In further consideration for the payment of sum (above stated) PATIENT agrees to refrain from directly or indirectly publishing or airing commentary upon DOCTOR and his practice, background, expertise and/or treatment — the sole exceptions being communication to a confidential dental-peer review body; to another healthcare provider; to a licensed attourney; to a governmental agency; in the context of a legal proceeding; or unless mandated by law. Publishing is intended to include attribution by name, by pseudonym, or anonymously. If PATIENT has prepared or does prepare commentary for publication about DOCTOR in violation of this agreement, the PATIENT (a) agrees to remove such commentary from publication or public display; and (b) exclusively assigns all Intellectual Property rights, including copyright(s), to DOCTOR for any written, pictorial, and/or electronic commentary.

If PATIENT violates this Confidentiality Agreement, PATIENT shall pay DOCTOR liquidated damages in the sum of Ten Thousand and no/100 Dollars.

I don't think so. The *Age of Reason* is gone. This is the *Age of Accountability*. He needs to think about this and learn from it. I do not want this to happen to any other PATIENT. All of this could have been avoided. Yes, it was my fault that I took the clindamycin; I trusted this DDS MSD to give me a safe and appropriate antibiotic. If I had had my wits about me I would have declined. My bad. However, clindamycin HCl is a broad-spectrum antibiotic that is to be used as a "last resort" to treat an infection that hasn't responded to other antibiotics. I didn't have an infection. THEN, he told me over the phone on Christmas Day to take Imodium and that he didn't think that I had *C. difficile* because of its rarity. That was wrong. Imodium could have killed me. Fortunately, by that time, I'd done some research and knew that taking the Imodium would have shut down the movement in my colon and could have easily resulted in Toxic Megacolon. This was his mistake and this really frightens me because it puts his patients in danger.

Clostridium difficile Testing:
http://labtestsonline.org/understanding/analytes/cdiff/tab/test

Went to Doc in the Box for the retesting paperwork to take to the lab.

EMAIL
From: Giorgi Namgaladze
<mailbox@phagetherapycenter.com>
Date: Sat, Feb 21, 2015 at 7:15 PM
Subject: RE: *Clostridium difficile*
To: esp <espbooks@gmail.com>

Dear Ellen,

With intestinal infections, usually not necessary to come to Georgia.

There are two types of E.coli, in terms of their toxicity:
- pathogenic E.coli, which produces toxins, sometimes very dangerous toxins. Commonly found in persons with dysbiosis.
- non-pathogenic E.coli, which is a good bacteria and necessary to have in the intestines for proper digestion. The non-pathogenic strains of E.coli produces enzyme that can usually reduce or kill off C.difficile.

The non-pathogenic E.coli is contained in capsule form, in combination with a number of other strains of probiotic bacteria - not a fecal transplant.

Again, we cannot guarantee successful treatment as there are no therapeutic phages for treating C.difficile.

With best regards,
Giorgi

http://en.wikipedia.org/wiki/Dysbiosis

Dysbiosis (also called dysbacteriosis) refers to microbial imbalance on or inside the body.[1] Dysbiosis is most commonly reported as a condition in the digestive tract. It has been associated with illnesses, such as inflammatory bowel disease[3],[4][5] chronic fatigue syndrome,[6] obesity,[7][8] cancer[9][10] and colitis.[11]

http://en.wikipedia.org/wiki/List_of_strains_of_Escherichia_coli

E. coli ~ Innocuous:

- Escherichia coli strain Nissle 1917 also known as Mutaflor

http://en.wikipedia.org/wiki/Mutaflor

Mutaflor®

http://mutaflor.ca/cart/

http://medfutures.com/portfolio/mutaflor/

Can't find any for sale in the USA or Canada.

http://www.healingwell.com/community/default.aspx?f=38&m=2673135 **Forum ~ Canada Halting Mutaflor**

http://mutaflor.ca/modes-of-action/

http://www.probiotics-help.com/mutaflor.html

References

http://www.karger.com/Article/Abstract/71488

Oral Administration of Probiotic *Escherichia coli* after Birth Reduces Frequency of Allergies and Repeated Infections Later in Life (after 10 and 20 Years)

Natural cure for *CDIFF* ~ Olive Leaf Extract

What is a natural cure for *CDIFF* bacterial infection?

Safety of Probiotic *Escherichia coli* Strain Nissle 1917 Depends on Intestinal Microbiota and Adaptive Immunity of the Host

Looks like Mutaflor® is off the market here in the USA and in Canada. Germany may have some for sale.

This book is for sale on Amazon:
E.coli: Probiotic for Piglet Diarrhoea: Escherichia Coli K88+ post Weaning Diarrhoea Paperback – May 26, 2008
by Amit Setia and Dr. Denis O. Krause

Probiotic bacteria could help treat Crohn's disease
Journal Reference:

1. C. Huebner, Y. Ding, I. Petermann, C. Knapp, L. R. Ferguson. **The Probiotic Escherichia coli Nissle 1917 Reduces Pathogen Invasion and Modulates Cytokine Expression in Caco-2 Cells Infected with Crohn's Disease-Associated *E. coli* LF82**. *Applied and Environmental Microbiology*, 2011; 77 (7): 2541 DOI: 10.1128/AEM.01601-10

American Society for Microbiology. "Probiotic bacteria

could help treat Crohn's disease." ScienceDaily. ScienceDaily, 1 April 2011. http://www.sciencedaily.com/releases/2011/03/110331142221.htm

The diarrhea stopped after I started drinking the black tea. I was lucky. I have tried to replenish, encourage, and nurture the good gut flora with food, herbs, supplements and probiotics. By continuing my whole food, plant-based diet I believe my risk of relapse or recurrence is minimized. However, if I put things into my mouth that could cause issues, it may result in a relapse of colitis. With time, my colon will heal and such diligence may not be as necessary. But for now I intend to put only good, healthy food into my body. Food is medicine.

If I were still having symptoms I would go the direction of the *E. coli* non-pathogenic treatment. Fecal Transplants do not interest me. Perhaps if the *E. coli* didn't work, I might consider the fecal transplant therapy. Maybe. I read that it has worked for many persons with Ulcerative Colitis (UC). The time could come when I might try anything but I am not up for this yet: http://www.naturalnews.com/037709_fecal_matter_c_diff_infection.html

22 FEBRUARY, SUNDAY *102.4 naked*

The words of kindness are more healing to a drooping heart than balm or honey. — Sarah Fielding

Good morning Sweetie Sunshine

I have been emailing with The Phage Therapy Center in Tbilisi, Georgia about *Clostridium difficile* phages. They don't have any available yet.

However, they use non-pathogenic *E. coli*, which are *C. difficile* antagonists, to control and/or kill the *C. difficile* bacteria. They have been using it for 80 years throughout the world, especially Europe (Germany & Georgia). It works for many gut issues including diverticulitis. Non-pathogenic *E. coli* is commonly in our good gut flora.

There was a product called Mutaflor® sold in Canada and USA but as of 2013 it was pulled and banned by the FDA.

This is so interesting.

I'm still taking enzymes and lots of probiotics. Yesterday I had a Chocolate Almond bar from CVS that boasted 20 billion CFUs of probiotics. Unfortunately it wasn't dairy-free. I let Claudio finish it off.

The dentist offered my money back if i don't sue and keep my mouth shut. I have to read the paperwork before I make a decision.

I am recovering but not gaining any weight. This has really been an ordeal and I am so glad that none of you got it. I read yesterday that some strains are not infectious. YIPPPEEEE

I am so ready for this to be over.

~ yoMama
END EMAIL

The best way to help your body protect itself against Ebola (or any virus or bacteria)
http://www.naturalnews.com/047232_Ebola_natural_immunit

23 FEBRUARY, MONDAY *103 pounds*
EDIT

Don't eat anything your great-grandmother wouldn't recognize as food. — Michael Pollan

Prebiotics
http://en.wikipedia.org/wiki/Prebiotic_%28nutrition%29
Prebiotics is a general term to refer to chemicals that induce the growth and/or activity of **commensal** microorganisms (e.g., bacteria and fungi) that contribute to the well-being of their host. The most common example is in the gastrointestinal tract, where prebiotics can alter the composition of organisms in the gut **microbiome**.

Sources
Chicory root is considered the richest natural source. Other traditional dietary sources of prebiotics include beans, Jerusalem artichoke, jicama, raw oats, unrefined wheat, unrefined barley, and yacon. Some of the oligosaccharides that naturally occur in breast milk are believed to play an important role in the development of a healthy immune system in infants.[13]

I feel pretty good today and will be buying some chicory tea for a prebiotic. I know of a coffee alternative that lists chicory root as a main ingredient. Perhaps this will be my new love. I eat a lot of beans, garlic, onion, asparagus, and bananas, but none other of the listed prebiotics.

Top 10 Foods Containing Prebiotics

Food	Prebiotic Fiber Content by Weight

115

Raw, Dry <u>Chicory</u> Root	64.6%
Raw, Dry <u>Jerusalem Artichoke</u>	31.5%
Raw, Dry <u>Dandelion</u> Greens	24.3%
Raw, Dry Garlic	17.5%
Raw, Dry <u>Leek</u>	11.7%
Raw, Dry Onion	8.6%
Raw <u>Asparagus</u>	5%
Raw <u>Wheat bran</u>	5.00%
Whole <u>Wheat flour</u>, Cooked	4.8%
Raw Banana	1%

Source:[14]

CHICORY ~ *Chichorium intybus L.*, root, leaf, ... Roots and leaves approved in Germany for treatment of loss of appetite and dyspepsia.
— *Peterson Field Guides, Western Medicinal Plants and Herbs,*
Steven Foster and Christopher Hobbs

The Maryland Law office is offering free consultations and they do cover California.

Here's a list of issues to discuss:

1. Imodium - contraindicative

2. Agreement - dentist

3. Publishing my journal

My sense is that I do not have a case because the periodontist recommended the Imodium in a phone conversation. It's his word against mine and he probably plays golf with members of the local judicial boy's club. Maybe we could subpoena the NSA to give us the recorded phone conversation for evidence? That would work.

Study reveals how *C. difficile* disrupts the gut
http://www.medicalnewstoday.com/articles/289817.php

Bugs in the System
http://www.economist.com/news/science-and-technology/21565586-bacterial-medicine-starting-emerge-bugs-system

I buy a little olive tree, pick and nibble on the baby soft leaves daily. In my garden I have oregano, peppermint, garlic, onions, potatoes, borage, thyme, parsley, comfrey, rosemary, dill, sage, chives, sweet potatoes, tomatoes, and wild strawberries. I often go outside to nibble.

~ LAWSUIT? ~

24 FEBRUARY, TUESDAY *104 pounds (after breakfast)*

I want the periodontist to learn from this mistake and not repeat it. I would like him to be more conscientious about handing out preventative antibiotics, especially the broad-spectrum ones like clindamycin HCl. And if he does, allow time to read the inserts and discuss this issue with patients letting them know the risk that they are taking. And if patients choose to take antibiotics, the DDS should always recommend taking probiotics to replace and re-colonize the intestinal bacteria that will be killed. And DO NOT RECOMMEND IMODIUM OR ANOTHER ANTI-DIARRHEAL MEDICATION WITHOUT TESTING FOR CLOSTRIDIUM DIFFICILE.

Am I being naïve hoping that he will learn from this lesson as much as I have? Or is it all about the $$?

I am feeling pretty good today. Except for lack of strength, my "energy" is 100%! I am back. I am in my body and my body is feeling good.

I drive to Monterey to pick up the stool sample containers from Quest Diagnostics, go to the library, Pharmaca, Trader Joe's, SaveMart, Cornucopia, Ace Hardware and home. BIG DAY for me going solo.

Had an interesting talk with Katie at Trader Joe's. Her daughter was in the Peace Corps in Nicaragua and caught MRSA. She had big lumps that would pop and leave holes on her body. Then she gave it to her boyfriend. Katie brought her daughter home, put her in intensive care and she almost died. I asked Katie if she'd write a piece for this book or write her own book about it. People have got to hear about this. As we were talking a lady jumps in to tell her story about an antibiotic-induced illness that almost killed her.

I have also asked LEENDA to write about her mom and her stay in nursing homes and probably had *CDIFF*. I've asked another friend whose mother is in a nursing home on the East Coast.

An older man in Pharmaca was looking at probiotics and we struck up a conversation about GMO wheat and GMO food in general. People want to talk.

I didn't find any Jerusalem artichokes but brought home a coffee alternative made from carob, barley, chicory and dandelion: Hazelnut flavor, Teeccino.com.

Bought a new probiotic from Pharmaca:
Dr. Ohhira's Probiotics Professional Formula
http://www.EssentialFormulas.com ~ took one right away.
Package info: Proprietary Fermented Culture - fermented culture medium of fruits vegetables, mushrooms and seaweeds containing naturally occurring lactic acid bacteria, prebiotics, enzymes, bacteriocins and trace amounts of vitamins, minerals and amino acids. Proprietary Lactic Acid Bacteria Blend 600 million CFU. Ingredients are fermented and processed for five years using 12 strains of lactic acid bacteria. All strains may not be present in final product. 100% vegetarian. Contains no dairy or gluten. Non-GMO, chemical-free. Product of Japan. Refrigeration not required.

I also bought a *Plant-Based VegaOne® All-in-One Nutritional Shake* French Vanilla flavor, Gluten-free, no sugar added, http://www.myvega.com. I first found this last Summer on my month-long backpacking trip.

I'm sparkling again, feeling good.

Claudio and I were just talking. I was relating Katie's story about her daughter giving MRSA to her boyfriend. Claudio expressed a fear of kissing me so I keyworded **C. diff kissing** and this came in:

https://answers.yahoo.com/question/index?
qid=20070615223828AAyuzLD

My Mother was just diagnosed with *C-diff* can she spread it to my father through kissing and cooking for him?

You don't have to worry about "catching" *Clostridium difficile*. Most of us already have it in our bowels, where it does no harm under normal circumstances.

****

[**NOT TRUE!!** I read that only 2 - 5% persons have C. difficile in their gut.] *C. difficile* may become established in the human colon; it is present in 2 – 5% of the adult population.[2] http://en.wikipedia.org/wiki/Clostridium_difficile_%28bacteria%29

**I

am happy. I am re-reading *The Starch Solution* by Dr. John McDougall to learn all that I can learn. I LOVE my diet. Claudio was not satisfied with answers.yahoo.com so I check another website:

http://www.webmd.com/digestive-disorders/news/20080530/c-diff-epidemic-what-you-must-know

C. diff **Epidemic: What You Must Know**

Why *C. diff* Is Spreading, Why It's More Deadly, How to Protect Your Family

http://www.webmd.com/digestive-disorders/news/20080530/c-diff-epidemic-what-you-must-know

WebMD.com *C. diff* Directory:

http://www.webmd.com/digestive-disorders/c-diff-directory

Slideshow Top Foods With Probiotics
http://www.webmd.com/digestive-disorders/probiotics-15/slideshow-probiotics
Yogurt, sauerkraut, miso, soft cheeses, kefir, sourdough bread, milk with probiotics (acidophilus), sour pickles (w/out vinegar), tempeh, probiotic supplements, prebiotics (asparagus, Jerusalem artichokes, bananas, oatmeal, red wine, honey, maple syrup, and legumes)

25 February, Wednesday *103.8 pounds*

And, of course, the funniest food of all, kumquats.
— George Carlin

Aloe, Swanson's probiotic, Teeccino® w/soy milk, VegaOne nutritional shake w/soy milk, banana, 3 rice cakes.

I feel good. I produce my stool sample for lab testing, get dressed and take it in. I meet Claudio in Carmel to have a birthday lunch for a friend, a great artist that Claudio has known since WAY back when in the old REAL Carmel ART days. I did not know he is a Pisces.

I make it through lunch. Claudio and I take a Carmel Beach walk of a little over two miles. Gassy Gut joins me and I flash back to the diarrhea when flatulence meant messy panties. I am afraid.

All goes well. I feel pretty good for my first real walk in the real world. Every day I shall exercise to gain

121

my strength back.

Beet salad w/pomegranate dressing, Dr. Ohhira's probiotic, aloe, green juice, almond meal, Teeccino tea, potatoes.

26 FEBRUARY, THURSDAY 102.6 pounds

The time indeed is at hand when systematic lectures on food will be part of medical education, when the value of feeding in disease is admitted to be as important as the administration of medicines.
— John Milner Fothergill

Feeling good again this morning. Took an award-winning, blue ribbon poo! Claudio was not amused but none-the-less happy for me.

27 FEBRUARY, FRIDAY 103 pounds

Ask not what you can do for your country. Ask what's for lunch.
— Orson Welles

Banana, coffee, Teeccino, toast w/jam, black Beluga lentils w/brown rice, tahini, solar baked sweet potato.

I put in a GoogleAlerts for clindamycin and thinking of starting a website for listing the *difficile*, phage and clindamycin GoogleAlerts that I receive.

http://www.dailyecho.co.uk/news/11824286.Killer_infections

<u>at hospital slashed by a smartphone app/</u>
MicroGuide was created by a team of Southampton General Hospital doctors to give patients bedside info on how to stop infections like *C.diff*

I make a website to keep track of new Internet articles that arrive as a result of my GoogleAlerts:
http://www.CDIFFbook.com

28 FEBRUARY, SATURDAY *104 pounds*

The body becomes what the foods are, as the spirit becomes what the thoughts are. — Kemetic Saying

EMAIL
On Sat, Feb 28, 2015 at 11:52 AM,
To: gnamgaladze@phagetherapycenter.com
esp <espbooks@gmail.com> wrote:
Thank you Giorgi

I am recovering!!! And very happy about it.

In my Internet research, these links say that Dr. Clokie has discovered phages for : **Bacteria-eating viruses 'magic bullets in the war on superbugs'**
https://www2.le.ac.uk/offices/press/press-releases/2013/october/bacteria-eating-viruses-2018magic-bullets-in-the-war-on-superbugs2019
University of Leicester

podcast:
https://soundcloud.com/university-of-leicester/martha-clokie-superbugs

http://www.leicestermercury.co.uk/Leicester-university-scientists-make-hospital/story-19941276-detail/story.html

Is this for real????

I have provided another stool sample to the lab for testing. I feel that it will not detect the Toxigenic *Clostridium difficile*.

I will let you know. I would think that if I had Toxigenic C. DIFF then I would have symptoms. I do not. I also know that CDI may recur.

best regards to you et al,
Ellen Pendleton

END EMAIL

This just came from the GoogleAlerts and I AM SO GLAD THAT I DIDN'T READ IT SOONER!!!!! I MIGHT HAVE FELT FEAR:

http://www.cdc.gov/HAI/organisms/cdiff/Cdiff_infect.html
from the CDC: ***Clostridium difficile* infection**

People getting medical care can catch serious infections called healthcare-associated infections (HAIs). One type of HAI – caused by the germ *C. difficile* – was estimated to cause almost half a million infections in the United States in 2011, and 29,000 died within 30 days of the initial diagnosis. Those most at risk are people, especially older adults, who take antibiotics and also get medical care. CDC provides guidelines and tools to the healthcare community to help prevent *Clostridium difficile* infections as well as provides resources to help the public safeguard their own health.

HOLY CRAP!!!!

124

"Shall we try a walk?" Claudio asks, having his own health issues with his knees, eager to field test them and me.

It is a gorgeous day here on the Big Sur Coast with welcomed rain this morning and it could rain again. Air temp is pleasant, not at all cold. And my body feels awesome. "Sure. How about a neighborhood walk?" I get out of my bathrobe.

We head out the door. I'm not quite sure how I'll do but I feel 100% today; weak for lack of exercise but capable and ready to rumble.

Spring is springing, mushrooms are popping out, creeks flowing, flowers blossoming and blooming. The woods smell sweet after the rain. It is a perfect day.

A little deer trail invites me up for an adventure. Oh Practical One advises otherwise. I stay on the manmade road. We pass the point where Scout and I had turned around. I'm feeling great.

Claudio has lived in this neighborhood for about 45 years. We walk by houses that we looked at when he was buying the one we're in now. We walk up, into the quiet. I check in with my body: Heart good, breathing great, muscles doing fine, gut happy. All is well.

After an hour or so we find ourselves up above the road we came in on and see it down below. "Can we get there from here cutting through the woods?" saving us time. We look for a cut-off trail but don't find one without poison oak and go back the way we came.

We stop at the house he lived in 40 years ago. The ocean view is the best. I take lots of photos. Claudio transitions into a younger self telling stories of living here for many years. "This is what I'd wake up to, seeing the waves crash on the rocks and this stretch of the horizon. Sunsets here are amazing."

Now I understand his propensity for a room with a view. I imagine waking up here every morning and my spirit delights.

We walk and return home after two or three hours. It wasn't a strenuous, huge walk but rather a leisurely stroll. I feel pleased that I did well. Nice.

3 MARCH, TUESDAY
BACK ON THE TRAIL

Children must be taught how to think, not what to think.
— Margaret Mead

I've spent the last couple days getting this ready for publication. Lots of work to do.

I'm feeling brave and Soberanes calls. Claudio has kept up on his hiking even through his knee issues, saying his knees feel best when he's hiking Soberanes. Today I join him and let him go up the trail first. Soberanes is the trail where we first met sixteen years ago. It is my training trail for backpacking and a spiritual place for us overlooking the beautiful Pacific Ocean and coastline.

We head up and I give attention to every moment willing to stop if necessary. But all systems are go.

"Welcome back," my partner chimes in.

"Good to be back. I missed you, Soberanes," and we hike up. Soberanes climbs from Highway 1 sea level straight up to 1000 feet in one mile. It's a great, fast workout full of incredible beauty. The spring wildflowers are beginning to bloom. The California golden poppies are gorgeous. The year that Claudio and I met up here was in the fall and it was the year of the Elegant Clarkia wildflowers, gorgeous red/purple covered the hillsides. The lupine are beginning to show now.

I am doing great, much to my surprise and much to Claudio's surprise too. I easily keep up.

We stop halfway up for water and Claudio says, "That's enough."

"Water?"

"No, walking. You've done great but I don't want to push it. This is far enough."

"Okay. You're probably right. I feel awesome! This is just what I needed."

"I'm so happy."

We turn around and go back down. I am in training for backpacking season! Hallelujah!!! I take lots of pictures and see whales spouting out to sea. *Thank you, Beautiful Body, for healing so well. namaste.*

We don't need a law against McDonald's or a law against slaughterhouse abuse — we ask for too much salvation by legislation. All we need to do is empower individuals with the right philosophy and the right information to opt out en masse.

— Joel Salatin

<u>CDC Says Deadly C. Difficile Bug May Be Transmitted Through Doctors' And Dentists' Offices</u>
<u>http://www.ibtimes.com/cdc-says-deadly-c-difficile-bug-may-be-transmitted-through-doctors-dentists-offices-1828970</u>

Doc in the Box calls. The Toxigenic C. DIFF was not detected but the antibody (produced by my body) is present. "How are you feeling?" Timothy asks.

"I am having some gut issues this morning."

"We would like to prescribe Flagyl," he says.

"So, my body is producing the C. DIFF antibody?"

"Yes, and it will show up in tests for years," Timothy tells me.

My body is fighting it. GOOD BODY! "I do not want to take the Flagyl. Will you send the test results to me?"

"Yes, we will mail them today."

(They do not want me to come into the office to pick them up.)

****

<u>http://www.naturalnews.com/048878 Liyfbiotic probiotics Je</u>

The non-GMO, powdered probiotic you've been waiting for: laboratory verified and based on Jerusalem Artichoke

EMAIL

Hello again Dearly Beloved

Only days after finishing the *CDIFF* book, i had some gut issues this morning. It might have been the coffee. *Damn! No mas.*

DocNBox called with my lab tests and the tests did not detect the Toxigenic *CDIFF at all.* GOOD! The *CDIFF* antibody showed up, which is also good and no *CDIFF* bacteria. They then recommended a round of Flagyl, another antibiotic. I refused.

The reason for publishing my book isn't to cure and heal people or to sell books (although these would be sweet bi-products) but rather to increase awareness for the *CDIFF* bacteria and hopefully prevent some unsuspecting person from going through what I did.

So if you know anyone who is going in for any kind of surgery, send them the link: *www.CDIFFbook.com.* A new video came out today and I posted it in the "I Read the News Today, Oh Yeah" section of the *CDIFF* webpage. Please pass it on to whomever you wish. I'd like to line up some radio interviews to speak up and speak out. Humph.

Claudio has a business associate who was hung up for a year with CDI symptoms. Initially he went into the hospital for hip surgery. The *CDIFF* almost killed him. This is not uncommon.

I have been very lucky and quite aware that relapses are typical. I am not outta the woods yet (rare for me to wanna get outta the woods, eh?). Even if you don't buy the book, please send the *www.CDIFFbook.com* webpage out there into the world. I don't want this to happen to another Spirit Being Human. HAPPY DAY to you.

PS ~ Jerusalem artichokes are an excellent prebiotic

END EMAIL

7 March, Saturday 102.8
Reaching Out

Aloe, TJs Green Juice, banana, avocado, oatmeal (almond meal, cinnamon, stevia, flaxseed meal), *Teeccino Herbal Coffee* (Gluten-free Dandelion Dark Roast) w/soy milk and stevia. No caffeine. Lentil & Brown Rice Bake, Yukon Gold potatoes dipped in tahini. Yum.

Luis Fábregas: Think twice about antibiotics — they enable killer superbug
http://triblive.com/opinion/luisfabregas/7899074-74/antibiotics-infection-diff#axzz3Tih2UKAJ

Sipping my second cup of *Teeccino Herbal Coffee* (caffeine-free) Dandelion Dark Roast this morning. I am in love. Good for me and good tasting. Perfect. I wonder if tea companies sponsor people like Nike® sponsors athletes?

http://www.naturalmedicinalherbs.net/herbs/c/ceratonia-siliqua=carob.php
Herb: Carob
Latin name: Ceratonia siliqua
Family: Leguminosae

I read the medicinal uses. I'm in. Now to find what carob looks like. Got it. It's a tree and I've seen them before. Now to find some Jerusalem artichokes. What do they look like? Roots! Lemme find some seeds and grow my own since I can't find them in local stores. Lemme look in my gardening books. Hours of enertainment.

Namaste.

8 MARCH, SUNDAY 102.8 pounds
THE LETTER TO THE DENTIST

Aloe w/Green Juice, hash brown potatoes w/hot sauce, Kevita, Teeccino, . . . no caffeine.

In putting the letter together I find out more about using the non-pathogenic *E. coli* for colitis, especially ulcerative colitis:

Maintaining remission of ulcerative colitis with the probiotic *Escherichia coli* Nissle 1917 is as effective as with standard mesalazine

http://www.ncbi.nlm.nih.gov/pmc/articles/PMC1774300/

Too bad we can't get Mutaflor® in the USA or Canada. Why can't we?????

9 MARCH, MONDAY

No caffeine. I spent yesterday putting together the reply letter to the dentist. I haven't finished yet. One thing I don't have is the insert for clindamycin. I intended to go to Pharmaca today, get one, and enclose it in the envelope with the letter. But I am impatient. So this morning I'm trying to find it online. I find this one with a big WARNING box on the webpage:

131

Clindamycin Hydrochloride: Package Insert and Label Information

http://druginserts.com/lib/rx/meds/clindamycin-hydrochloride-31/#w-box

WARNING BOX on insert:

Clostridium difficile associated diarrhea (CDAD) has been reported with use of nearly all antibacterial agents, including clindamycin hydrochloride and may range in severity from mild diarrhea to fatal colitis. Treatment with antibacterial agents alters the normal flora of the colon, leading to overgrowth of *C. difficile*.

Because clindamycin hydrochloride therapy has been associated with severe colitis which may end fatally, it should be reserved for serious infections where less toxic antimicrobial agents are inappropriate, as described in the <u>INDICATIONS AND USAGE</u> section. It should not be used in patients with nonbacterial infections such as most upper respiratory tract infections.

C. difficile produces toxins A and B, which contribute to the development of CDAD. Hypertoxin producing strains of *C. difficile* cause increased morbidity and mortality, as these infections can be refractory to antimicrobial therapy and may require colectomy. CDAD must be considered in all patients who present with diarrhea following antibiotic use. Careful medical history is necessary since CDAD has been reported to occur over two months after the administration of antibacterial agents.

If CDAD is suspected or confirmed, ongoing antibiotic use not directed against *C. difficile* may need to be discontinued. Appropriate fluid and electrolyte management, protein supplementation, antibiotic treatment of *C. difficile*, and surgical evaluation should be instituted as clinically indicated.

Why didn't I read this before I popped those pills into my mouth? Do I have to learn the hard way? (I forgive myself.) I wonder if the periodontist I went to has read this WARNING BOX?????

The rest of the insert is here:
http://druginserts.com/lib/rx/meds/clindamycin-hydrochloride-31/

http://druginserts.com/lib/rx/meds/clindamycin-hydrochloride-31/page/2/#indications

An Internet article just arrived from LA Times:
http://www.dailynews.com/health/20150305/these-robots-kill-germs-at-southern-california-hospitals
These robots kill germs at Southern California hospitals
In five minutes, Merlin sends out 450 pulses of ultra-violet light that flash against walls, the bed, the counter and sink to obliterate the drug-resistant staph bacteria, knock out *Clostridium difficile* spores and erase any hint of the measles.

Perfect! Can I be in the room too??? Many years ago I wrote about The Strecker Memorandum and eradicating HIV in humans with electromagnetic frequencies and learning how to produce healing frequencies via meditation. My research project is now. Through all of this I have been meditating. However, the quality of my meditation was compromised using caffeine, so I would meditate early in the morning pre-caffeine. Now I am caffeine-free so off we go.

The healing theory is that when we meditate our brainwave frequency changes and permeates throughout the body. Dr. David R. Hawkins wrote a book: Power vs. Force, and has a chart giving a frequency value of various emotions from shame to enlightenment. Manfred Clynes invented a device to record emotions through the

fingertips and music:
http://en.wikipedia.org/wiki/Manfred_Clynes
and this:
http://www.angelfire.com/ca3/espbooks/Clynes.html

Teeccino this morning, Herbal Coffee Alternative, Hazelnut 75% organic, buttery hazelnuts enriched by golden roasted almonds, slighty sweet from dates & figs. Medium Roast, all-purpose grind. 11 oz. It's ground like coffee and uses a cone and filter (pretend coffee). Ingredients: Carob, Barley, Chicory root, dates, figs, almonds, natural flavors. I add stevia and soy milk. Prebiotics. Yummy. It's making a nice transition to coffee-free.

10 MARCH, TUESDAY
TEST RESULTS

Caffeine-free. I finish my letter to DDS, photocopy and get it ready it for the post office.

LETTER
Dear DDS,

I am still recovering.

I have lived to learn valuable lessons from this experience and it is my hope that you will too.

1. Please do not prescribe clindamycin as a preventative. Please do not offer clindamycin to unsuspecting patients without reading out loud with them the side effects on the insert. *Clostridium difficile* infection is on the rise and in 2011 *Clostridium difficile* killed almost 29,000 persons in the USA. If I had read the insert prior to procedure I would not have taken it. My bad.

****

Clindamycin Hydrochloride: Package Insert and Label Information
http://druginserts.com/lib/rx/meds/clindamycin-hydrochloride-31/#w-box
WARNING
Clostridium difficile associated diarrhea (CDAD) has been reported with use of nearly all antibacterial agents, including clindamycin hydrochloride and may range in severity from mild diarrhea to fatal colitis. Treatment with antibacterial agents alters the normal flora of the colon, leading to overgrowth of *C. difficile*.

http://druginserts.com/lib/rx/meds/clindamycin-hydrochloride-31/page/2/#indications
Because of the risk of colitis, as described in the WARNING box, before selecting clindamycin hydrochloride capsules, USP, the physician should consider the nature of the infection and the suitability of less toxic alternatives (e.g., erythromycin).
****

2. Imodium. I stopped taking the clindamycin after 12 capsules (out of 21). My *gut feeling* was that it was not good for me. On Christmas Day when I told you about the symptoms, diarrhea, weight loss, fatigue and the *Clostridium difficile* suspicion, you recommended black tea

and Imodium. The black tea stopped the diarrhea but I said that I would not take the Imodium because I had read not to take it with the suspected presence of *Clostridium difficile*. You said, "I doubt that you have C. difficile. It is very rare." This was your bad. The next day I went to Doctors on Duty and the stool samples detected Toxigenic *C. difficile*.

****

Four Mistakes that lead to *C. Difficle* Lawsuits
https://www.millerandzois.com/four-mistakes-that-lead-to-c-difficle-lawsuits.html

C. difficile has bedeviled hospitals for years. The number of *C. difficile* cases in this country has risen and so have the number of medical malpractice cases involving *C. difficile*. One common problem is the continued use of anti-peristaltic medications like **Imodium or Lomotil**. Both are contraindicated so if a doctor sees signs and symptoms that the patient might have *C. diff*, the doctors must stop prescribing that medication.

****

Taking the Imodium could have led to Toxic MegaColon or death.

****

From the National Institute of Health
http://www.nlm.nih.gov/medlineplus/druginfo/meds/a682399.html

Clindamycin
pronounced as (klin" da mye' sin)

IMPORTANT WARNING:
Many antibiotics, including clindamycin, may cause overgrowth of dangerous bacteria in the large intestine. This may cause mild diarrhea or may cause a life-threatening condition called colitis (inflammation of the large intestine). Clindamycin is more likely to cause this type of infection than many other antibiotics, so it should only be used to treat serious infections that cannot be treated by

other antibiotics.
****

In my case I did not have an infection nor did we talk about clindamycin or discuss other options. Clindamycin should not be prescribed as a preventative to anyone. I should have done the homework and believe me, I will from now on.

****

CDC Says Deadly *C. Difficile* Bug May Be Transmitted Through Doctors' And Dentists' Offices

http://www.ibtimes.com/cdc-says-deadly-c-difficile-bug-may-be-transmitted-through-doctors-dentists-offices-1828970

ABC News Video:
http://abcnews.go.com/GMA/video/warning-cdiff-superbug-29239523 ~ **New CDC Warning About *CDIFF* Superbug**

http://www.cdc.gov/mmwr/preview/mmwrhtml/mm6109a3.htm
Vital Signs: Preventing *Clostridium difficile* Infections
Conclusions: Nearly all CDIs are related to various health-care settings where predisposing antibiotics are prescribed and *C. difficile* transmission occurs.

https://www.youtube.com/watch?v=Af5qUxl1ktI
The gut flora: You and your 100 trillion friends: Jeroen Raes at TEDxBrussels

http://www.cdph.ca.gov/programs/hai/Documents/2013-CDI-TechNotes_-02.02.15.pdf
TECHNICAL NOTES
***Clostridium difficile* Infections in California Hospitals, 2013**
Virtually all patients with *Clostridium difficile* Infection (CDI) received antibiotics between two weeks and three months prior to the infection; therefore, judicious use of antibiotics is also important in decreasing and preventing CDI.

****

Your agreement cover letter reads: "In the spirit of putting this behind us, and with my greater concern that you spend your efforts on focusing on your health, ..." *I have spent all of my time since December 25 "focusing on my health" and trying to get well again. It has my complete attention, believe me. This was a big lesson for both of us. So "in the spirit of putting this behind us," I would still like a refund of $1622. In good faith I cannot sign such a restrictive agreement as you have presented.*

My intention is to educate the public regarding the subject of antibiotic-induced colitis, warning them from my experience. I've written a book about this, as my laptop and I had plenty of time together since Christmas.

At Doctors on Duty, an assistant delivers the diagnosis of **Toxigenic C. difficile detected** *and gives a prescription to me for Metronidazole/Flagyl. I refuse it, "I won't take it."*

"Why not?" the assistant asks.

I quote: Due to its potential carcinogenic properties, metronidazole is banned in the <u>European Union</u> and the <u>USA</u> for veterinary use in the feed of animals and is banned for use in any food animals in the USA.[22][23]

Metronidazole (Flagyl) ~
<u>http://en.wikipedia.org/wiki/Metronidazole</u>

The assistant leaves to talk with the doctor, then returns. In the waiting room full of sick people eagerly waiting

138

their turn with the doctor, the assistant starts yelling at me, "The doctor says that you'll end up in the hospital. You have to take it."

I didn't take it. I did not and will not take vancomycin or Fidaxomicin. No more antibiotics. I bought some probiotics. I have chosen to trust my inner guidance and my body to heal naturally with a strict, whole food plant-based vegan diet (no oil, no sugar), rest, probiotics, prebiotics, loving support and faith.

Regarding probiotics, I discovered specific probiotics that target C.DIFF and one that helps the CDI symptoms. These are in my book. I have also found that some non-pathogenic E. coli are C.DIFF antagonists, have been available in USA and Canada and are rather successful in eradicating C.DIFF. It is now banned in the USA and Canada barring very expensive lab testing requirements by the FDA/Big Pharma collusion. Mutaflor® is one brand of non-pathogenic E. coli and is available in Europe. http://www.probiotics-help.com/mutaflor.html

Bacteriophage research proves interesting and valuable. A phage for C.DIFF has possibly been discovered at the University of Leicester in the UK but is not ready for the public. It will take years to come to market.

In conclusion I would still like my money back, the $1622,

that I paid for this experience, even though my expenses, time and suffering far exceed this monetary value. My intention is to not mention or publish your name at all. If you can trust me then we can do this honorably with integrity. The agreement is lawyer stuff and they tend to get carried away. A lawyer has outlined my options and I would prefer to publish my book, inform the public of the risks involved in taking antibiotics and not mention your name. I will agree to not ask you for more money or sue you. [Exceptions: any Class Action Suits regarding clindamycin.] If this can work for you please let me know.

best regards,
Ellen Pendleton

PS ~ I will also email this letter with the active Internet links.
END LETTER

I received the lab results yesterday but I don't understand what it means: CLOSTRIDIUM DIFFICILE NOT ISOLATED. REFERENCE RANGE NOT ISOLATED. So I'm online trying to figure it out. Quest Diagnostics isn't giving me the latest results, let alone explain them.

http://www.ncbi.nlm.nih.gov/pmc/articles/PMC3147743/
Impact of Clinical Symptoms on Interpretation of Diagnostic Assays for *Clostridium difficile* Infections

This article is beyond me but has an impressive reference list to explore. Let me try again:

http://www.cdc.gov/HAI/organisms/cdiff/Cdiff_faqs_HCP.html

Frequently Asked Questions about *Clostridium difficile* for Healthcare Providers

Healthcare-associated Infections (HAIs)

This FAQ page carries a lot of information, especially regarding the different tests available for *C.DIFF*. I could have started here if I'd found it earlier.

Tracking *Clostridium difficile* Infection

http://www.cdc.gov/hai/organisms/cdiff/tracking-Cdiff.html

http://www.umassmed.edu/Global/Regional%20Science%20Resource%20Center/DecFocus2008%5B1%5D.pdf

Phase 2 trial shows promising results for *C. difficile* treatment

Donna Ambrosin, MD

Search didn't pull up anything for the keywords:

Donna Ambrosin *difficile*.

I have an appointment Thursday with Doc in the Box to find out what *C. DIFFICILE NOT ISOLATED* means.

I am eager to get this book out there and maybe reach someone who might need help regarding this subject.

DeBoles® organic Fettuccine pasta is made with Jerusalem artichoke Inulin. I buy some, cook it and it's now my favorite pasta.

www.deboles.com   ~ Organic Artichoke Inulin Pasta

DeBoles proudly offers the only brand of premium organic handmade pastas made with Jerusalem artichoke flour. A rich source of protein and dietary fiber as compared to traditional pasta, Jerusalem artichoke flour also naturally contains inulin, a prebiotic that stimulates the growth of beneficial bacterial in the digestive tract that in turn aids digestion and lowers blood pressure and cholesterol. Our signature recipe has a subtle nutty flavor and light smooth texture that is never sticky.

FOOD, GLORIOUS FOOD! I still haven't found any Jerusalem artichokes. Bought some Mocha caffeine-free Teeccino®, with carob, barley, chicory. Yum.

NOTE: In the beginning I logged my food intake rather diligently; I wanted to keep track. But as I started feeling better I got lazy and didn't log all the food that I would eat for that day. So some days just one or two food items are listed, for example, "Probiotics, banana, . . ." or "Coffee, aspirin, ..." These were the first foods of the day, then I'd stop logging. I eat a lot. On a whole food plant-based diet I eat all day long, letting my stomach digest in between for about 45 minutes to an hour. I keep steamed, small potatoes in my refrigerator for an easy snack. And I discovered that sunchokes is another name for Jerusalem artichokes. Now I can find them.

12 MARCH, THURSDAY *106 pounds*
ONE MORE TIME

I go to Doc in the Box. The person who called me with the test results the other day, is my doctor today. He walks into the room and talks to me like I am two years old, explaining gut flora. I let him talk, curious to know if I might learn more. He says that I am clean. They tried their best to grow the *C. difficile* bacteria in the lab from my stool sample but could not.

Then it is my turn. I tell him everything I've been through and learned since December 1. "I'm a journaler. My laptop and I were bedridden for two months and journaled the entire adventure."

He says, "I'd like to read it."

namaste

EMAIL TO KEVITA.COM

i just kicked *Clostridium difficile's* butt and found that your Blueberry Cherry Kevita was my preferred drink. Is it your only product with mangosteen?????

and thank you so much. I LOVE your products (especially w/stevia, not sugar) *grazie mille*
ellen pendleton
http://www.CDIFFbook.com
END EMAIL

[NOTE: Trader Joe's now sells Raw Shelled Hemp Seeds with 2.5g Omega-3, 8.5g Omega-6 and 10g of protein in a 3 tablespoon serving. And they taste GREAT!!!]

I find some sunchokes/Jerusalem artichokes and turmeric roots at Whole Foods. I peel the sunchokes and eat some. Yum. I peel and use the turmeric in a curry dish. A few of the sunchokes have new growth after a few days, so I plant them and a turmeric root. I hope they grow.

~ OMG ~

02 MAY, SATURDAY
A NEW FIND

. . . How much bondage and suffering a woman escapes when she takes the liberty of being her own physician of both body and soul.
— Elizabeth Cady Stanton

Claudio is having his Men's Group here next Wednesday through Sunday. The house needs to be fluffed and ready. I'm busy doing this. I have camping reservations at The Pinnacles National Park for five nights. In the process of cleaning my office to set up an AirBed, I find some paperwork from Doc in the Box from when I first went in for testing on 26 December 2014. I hadn't read it till now and it says on page 2:

MEDICATIONS ADMINISTERED
Loperamide [RxNorm: 978006], 2mg Capsules
2 caps now then 1 after each loose stool, no more than 4 per 24 hrts *(sp?)*

Then on page 3 it says:
FOLLOW-UP LABORATORY to be done include CBC w/ diff, comprehesive metabolic panel, stool O&P, stool culture, C. dificile,. *(sp)*

Loperamide is Imodium. Are they trying to kill us?

23 June, Wednesday
BRAT Diet Correction

In re-reading the information from the Doc in the Box paperwork, i see that the **BRAT** *diet equals Bananas, Rice, Applesauce, and Toast (not tea). I don't eat a lot of wheat so the tea worked for me. namaste.*

The sunchokes and turmeric are growing in my greenhouse. And I am done eating soy, corn, and other GMO suspects.

REFERENCES

Clindamycin Insert:
http://druginserts.com/lib/rx/meds/clindamycin-hydrochloride-31/

http://www.virginia.edu/uvaprint/HSC/pdf/08005.pdf
INFECTION PREVENTION & CONTROL
PATIENT INFORMATION SHEET
CLOSTRIDIUM DIFFICILE (C. diff)
PATIENT INFORMATION SHEET

Mutaflor® References:
http://www.probiotics-help.com/mutaflor.html

References
1.Mutaflor: The Probiotic Drug for Life: Inflammatory Bowel Disease and Chronic Functional Bowel Diseases, *Ardeypharm GmBH*, Germany

2.Kuzela L et al; Induction and Maintenance of Remission with Nonpathogenic Escherichia Coli in Patients with Pouchitis; *Am J Gastroenterol*; 2001;96:3218-3219

3.Kruis W et al.; Maintaining Remission of Ulcerative Colitis with the Probiotic Escherichia Coli Nissle 1917 is as Effective as with Standard Mesalazine; *Gut*; 2004, 53:1617-1623

4.Kruis W et al; Double-Blind Comparison of an Oral Escherichia Coli Preparation and Mesalazine in Maintaining Remission of Ulcerative Colitis, *Aliment Pharmacol Ther*; 1997; 11: 853-858

5.Rembacken, B. J; Non-Pathogenic Escherichia Coli versus Mesalazine for the Treatment of Ulcerative Colitis: a Randomised Trial; *Lancet*; 1999; 354: 635-639

6.Malchow HA; Crohn's Disease and Escherichia coli.; *J Clin Gastroenterol*; 1997; 25: 653-658

7.Goerg, K. J., et al.; <u>A New Approach in Pseudomembranous Colitis: Probiotic Escherichia coli Nissle 1917 After Intestinal Lavage</u>; *Eur J Gastroenterol Hepatol*; 2008; 20(2): 155-156

8.Fric, P., et al.; <u>The Effect of Non-Pathogenic Escherichia Coli in Symptomatic Uncomplicated Diverticular Disease of the Colon</u>; *Eur J Gastroenterol Hepatol* ; 2003; 15: 313-315

9.Henker, J.et al; <u>Probiotic Escherichia Coli Nissle 1917 versus Placebo for Treating Diarrhea of Greater than 4 Days Duration in Infants and Toddlers</u>; *Pediatr Infect Dis J* 2008; 27(6): 494-49

10.Bruckschen E et al; <u>Chronic Constipation. Comparison of Microbiological and Lactulose Treatment</u>; [German]; *MMW* 1994, 16: 241-245

11.Möllenbrink, M., et al; <u>Treatment of Chronic Constipation with Physiologic Escherichia Coli Bacteria. Results of a Clinical Study of the Effectiveness and Tolerance of Microbiological Therapy with the E. Coli Nissle 1917 strain (Mutaflor)</u> [German]; *Med Klin*; 1994, 89: 587-593

12.Plaßmann, D., et al; <u>Treatment of Irritable Bowel Syndrome with Escherichia Coli Strain Nissle 1917 (EcN): a Retrospective Survey</u>; *Med Klin 2007*; 102 (11): 888-892

RESOURCES

BOOKS, BY AUTHOR
Campbell, T. Colin, *The China Study,* BenBella Books, 10300 N. Central Expy., Suite 530, Dallas, TX 75231. 2006
Foster, Steven, Christopher Hobbs, *Western Medicinal Plants and Herbs, Peterson Field Guides,* Houghton Mifflin Harcourt
Hever, Julienna, *The Complete Idiot's Guide to Plant-based Nutrition*, Alpha Books, 800 East 96th Street, Indianapolis, IN 46240. 2011
McDougall, Dr. John, *The Starch Solution*, Rodale Books, 4300 Glendale Milford Road, Cincinnati, OH 45242. 2013
Mickel, Dr. David, *Chronic Fatigue Syndrome, ME and Fibromyalgia. The Long Awaited Cure,* New Generation Publishing. 2004

BOOKS, BY TITLE
Physicians Desk Reference of Medicinal Herbs, Thomson Reuters; 3 Times Square, New York, NY 10036 USA. 2007

VIDEOS
Forks Over Knives, Monica Beach Media, (323) 957-0730. 2011
Save Your Life Herbal Video Collection, Sam Biser, University of Natural Healing. http://www.sambiser.com

LINKS
Clostridium difficile, colitis, and phage news updates and videos: www.CDIFFbook.com
Ellen Pendleton, author, www.ellenpendleton.com
Resources4Healing, www.Resources4Healing.com
Whole Food Plant-Based Resources
www.angelfire.com/ca3/espbooks/plant-based.html
www.GrandmaCamping.com

*The Internet could be a very positive step towards
education, organization and participation in a
meaningful society.*
~ Noam Chomsky

*I'm just glad to be feeling better. I really thought
I'd be seeing Elvis soon.*
~ Bob Dylan

for you who open books from the back — Welcome!

150